Praise for Dr. Alterman and
HOW TO CONTROL DIABETES

"The patient's knowledge and understanding of diabetes is the cornerstone of treatment for this common but complex disease. Dr. Alterman has offered, in a comprehensible approach, the optimum methods for blood glucose control, rational choices of diets, and the role of exercise in reducing the risk of long-term complications of diabetes mellitus. I recommend it highly."
　　　—DAVID N. REINHARD, M.D., Chief
　　　Section of Endocrinology and Diabetes
　　　Miami Heart Institute

"Need an up-to-date popular book on living with diabetes? Neatly arranged and organized, this layperson's guide may fill the bill. Written in a kindly but not overly chummy manner and definitely for the mass audience, it includes a large glossary and plenty of lists. . . ."
　　　—*Booklist*

*Please turn the page
for more acclaim . . .*

"Dr. Seymour Alterman, a well-known diabetologist, has written a most helpful book for those afflicted with diabetes (Type I or Type II) and their families. Not only is this book informative but it is also a pleasure to read, easy to understand, and simple to follow. He covers both the cause and management of the disease and how to deal with the psychological problems that living with diabetes creates. I recommend the book to anyone who has been recently diagnosed as diabetic as well as those who have been living with it for years. They will find much new information that will make their life pleasanter, healthier, and more hopeful."

—DR. ALICE GINOTT, Ph.D., Psychology

HOW TO CONTROL DIABETES

A Complete Guide and Meal Planner to Live a Longer, Healthier, and Happier Life

**Seymour L. Alterman, M.D., F.A.C.P.
Edited by
Donald A. Kullman, M.D.**

BALLANTINE BOOKS • NEW YORK

Published by Ballantine Books

This publication is designed to provide accurate and authoritative information in regard to the subject matter covered. This book is not intended to replace the advice and guidance of a trained physician nor is it intended to encourage self-treatment of illness or medical disease. Diabetes is a life-threatening metabolic disorder and diabetic patients must seek counsel and instructions from their personal physician who is familiar with their individual case.

http://www.randomhouse.com

Library of Congress Catalog Card Number: 97-93876

ISBN 0-345-42158-2

This edition published by arrangement with Lifetime Books, Inc.

Manufactured in the United States of America

First Ballantine Books Edition: November 1997

10   9   8   7   6   5   4   3   2

Contents

Foreword   xi
Preface   xiii

1. *What Is Diabetes Mellitus?*   1
   Metabolic Disorder • History • Classifications

2. *Type I and Type II Diabetes:*
   Two Different Disorders   8
   Definitions • Characteristics • Ketoacidosis

3. *Gestational Diabetes (Diabetes and Pregnancy)*   19
   Incidence • Diagnosis • Management and
   Prognosis

4. *Guidelines for Healthier Eating*
   With Diabetes   26
   Importance for Diabetic Control • Exchange
   Lists • Meal Planning

5. *The Pritikin Program and Diabetes*   45
   Benefits of the Pritikin Program • The Pritikin
   Diet • Special Guidelines for Diabetics

6. *Insulin*   62
   Sources of Insulin • Different Types and Mode
   of Action • Cautions Regarding Use

7. *Preparing and Injecting Insulin*   **70**
    Insulin Syringes • Injection Sites • Antiseptic
    Techniques • Preparation of Mixture

8. *Self-Monitoring of Blood Glucose
    (SMBG) and Laboratory Testing
    for Glycosylated Hemoglobin*   **76**
    Finger-Stick Method • Glycosylated
    Hemoglobin • Equipment

9. *Hypoglycemia*   **84**
    Causes of Low Sugar Reactions • How to
    Recognize Hypoglycemia • Importance of Early
    Treatment • Comparison of Diabetic Coma and
    Insulin Reactions

10. *Oral Drugs for Diabetes*   **92**
    Indications for Use • Sulfonylureas •
    Biguanides

11. *Patterns of Control and Sick Day Care*   **102**
    Information Gleaned From Careful Records in
    Diary Form • Case Histories • Sick Day Rules

12. *Intensive Management of Diabetes*   **112**
    Effect on Vision • Renal Function • Nerve
    Tissue • Cardiovascular Disease

13. *The Insulin Pump*   **121**
    Advantages Over Conventional Treatment •
    Description of Equipment and Maintenance •
    Getting Started

14. *Obesity and the Diabetic*   **127**
    Importance of Weight Control • Practical
    Methods of Treatment • Dietary and Exercise
    Approach

15. *Benefits of Exercise*   **140**
    Beneficial Effects on Metabolism • Medical
    Clearance for Exercise • Appropriate Exercise
    Programs

16. *Diabetes, Lipids, and Atherosclerosis* **147**
Definition of "Good" and "Bad" Cholesterol •
Decreasing Risk of Cardiovascular Disease •
Newest Drugs for Treatment

17. *Long-Term Complications of Diabetes* **171**
Neuropathy • Cardiovascular Disease •
Retinopathy • Nephropathy

18. *Travel and the Diabetic* **193**
Planning a Trip • Equipment to Take When
Traveling • Necessary Precautions

19. *Hygiene* **198**
Dental Care • Skin Care • Foot Care • Eye Care •
Urinary Tract Infections

20. *Care of the Feet* **205**
How to Avoid Ulcers and Infections •
Importance of Early Diagnosis and Treatment •
Routine Foot Care

21. *Diabetes and Impotence* **214**
Physiologic and Psychologic Causes • Medical
Treatment • Surgical Treatment

22. *Straight Talk to Teenagers and Young
Adults With Diabetes* **221**
What to Tell Friends and Teachers • How to
Live a "Normal" Life • Answers to Questions
Frequently Asked by Young Diabetics

23. *Diabetes in Black Americans* **229**
Epidemiology of Diabetes in African Americans
• Need for Increased Awareness and Treatment •
U.S. Government Conferences

24. *Diabetes in Hispanics* **234**
High Incidence of Type II Diabetes • Challenge
for Hispanics • Spanish Language Publications

25. *The Psychology of Diabetes*   239
Denial and Rebellion • Anxiety and Depression
• Effects of Stress • Family's Role

26. *Hope for the Future*   245
Pancreatic and Kidney Transplant • Islet Cells
Transplantation • Animal Cures • Newest Drugs
• Genes That Affect Diabetes and Obesity

Glossary   253
Index   271

Foreword

In this most informative book, Dr. Alterman addresses the significant issues and vexing problems diabetics of all ages face on a daily basis.

The text, with its charts and clear guidelines, in HOW TO CONTROL DIABETES presents up-to-date and practical information which is vital for those who have diabetes and those who take care of them.

Dr. Alterman, an acknowledged authority in the field of diabetes and metabolic disorders, has written a book on diabetes that is clear, concise, and informative.

This book covers in an easy-to-understand but comprehensive manner a wide range of topics important to the diabetic. Dr. Alterman offers guidelines regarding management of diabetes at work, at play, and while traveling.

There is no doubt that in-depth knowledge and understanding of the disease processes are essential cornerstones in the treatment and control of this common but complex disorder.

This book reviews the best available techniques for monitoring blood glucose levels and outlines a rational approach to the nutritional needs of the diabetic. Dr. Alterman carefully explains the added role of regular exercise in helping the diabetic reduce the risk of short- and long-term complications and overcome insulin resistance.

Adopting better strategies for nutrition and exercise usually result in the better utilization of available insulin.

There are a multitude of books on diabetes available to the public. Most of these publications are either too elementary or too complex for the reader. Most of them contain dated material. Dr. Alterman's book is easy to read and understand. Technical terms are broken down and rephrased into simple terms. This book contains important up-to-date clinical and research information that is focused on the better control and eventual cure of diabetes.

I recommend it highly as a reference source for those primary care physicians who deal with diabetes and for most diabetics who need a "primer" to better understand the nature of the metabolic disorder with its difficult complications and sequelae. Many of these can be improved or even prevented by careful control of the blood sugar and restoration of the normal biochemical balance through improved nutrition, regular exercise and weight control, and, when indicated, drug intervention.

—ROBERT E. BAUER, M.D., A.A.C.P.
Senior Attending Physician
Mount Sinai Medical Center,
Miami Beach, Florida

Preface

DIABETES: THE EPIDEMIC AND THE CURE

Diabetes affects over seventeen million people in the United States, half of whom are completely unaware of their disorder. Diabetes may be asymptomatic for years. Notwithstanding, some patients fail to recognize the meaning of such early symptoms of diabetes as increased thirst and frequent urination, or they attribute them to the aging process. For many, medical care is not sought until the development of one of the long-term complications of diabetes—failing kidneys, eye or nerve damage—motivates treatment. This book will alert the reader to the steps he can take to prevent or delay these complications and will help him to assume a more active role in controlling his diabetes. Only through knowledge can the diabetic make informed choices to coincide with personal treatment goals and philosophy.

Much progress has been made in recent years. In the future it may be possible to administer insulin without injections, via patches or nasal sprays. Devices that can read the blood sugar without the necessity of having to prick the finger to get a blood sample are being developed. The most specific type of treatment for diabetes is transplantation of the pancreas or the insulin-producing islet cells. However, the susceptibility of transplanted tissue to rejection and the toxicity of the immunosuppressive drugs employed to prevent this from occurring have been the major biological barriers to this procedure. The islet cell transplant technique involves the injection of donor cells into the portal vein of the recipient, which carries them to the liver, where hopefully they will implant themselves in their new host and secrete insulin as needed. Many successful transplants have been performed. The insulin dose of the patient is usually reduced after a successful transplant, and some have been able to stop their insulin completely. However, there is a shortage of donor organs and the immunosuppressive drugs required to prevent rejection must be monitored carefully for potential significant side effects. The concomitant transplantation of bone marrow cells from the islet cell donor has recently proven effective in tricking the recipient's body into accepting the new islet cells as its own. This experimental protocol eliminates the need for antirejection medications.

The outlook for a cure for diabetes has never been brighter. Indeed, experimental cures in primates have already been accomplished. The technology has not yet been successfully applied to humans, but the rapid advances in laboratory research point to a human cure just around the corner. While we are waiting for a technological breakthrough, we must not neglect the cure that is already here for many diabetics—a disciplined program of diet, exercise, and weight loss. Until a permanent cure is found, every diabetic should regard his disorder as a slow and often silently progressive disease that takes its toll through the years because of chronically elevated blood sugars. The state-of-the-art measures described in this book can do much to keep the blood sugar under control and allow the diabetic to live a long and healthy life.

To appreciate the importance of these apparently simple measures in controlling diabetes, the plight of the Pima

Native Americans of Arizona serves as a microcosm of the general diabetic population. Fifty years ago the disease was unknown among these people. The dramatic rise in incidence has been attributed to the change in lifestyle and diet that has taken place during the past half century. A federal dam project rerouted rivers and flooded farmlands, depriving the Pimas of their basic source of food. A diet based upon fresh fruits and vegetables produced by physical labor was no longer available to these industrious people. Well-meaning government aid (in the form of highly processed fatty foods that were doled out without requiring any physical efforts on the part of the recipients) has produced disastrous results. Although the Pimas were born with the genes that predisposed them to the development of diabetes, their former lifestyle was sufficient to prevent the disease from manifesting itself. With the loss of their healthy protective diet and physical work activities, obesity has become commonplace and diabetes so prevalent that it threatens the very survival of this genetically susceptible population. The Pimas' plight clearly demonstrates what has long been known: diet, lifestyle, and obesity are major factors in precipitating Type II diabetes. The Pimas cannot change their genetic susceptibility, but like all diabetics they can take measures to control their disorder.

In spite of the fact that you may have inherited the gene that predisposed you to developing Type II diabetes, by changing your lifestyle and eating habits you can "cure" or dramatically reduce its effects.

In other words, many people with Type II diabetes who lose weight, watch their diet, and increase their level of physical activity do extremely well. Their bodies regain some of the lost sensitivity to insulin, and the quantity of insulin produced by their pancreas may once again suffice to meet their needs. If these individuals go off their diet, gain weight, and once again live a sedentary lifestyle, their blood sugar levels will most certainly rise and the diabetes will manifest itself once again. The measures suggested in this book are most effective when started early in the course of the disease. If there is a delay of ten or more years before instituting the changes set forth, you may lessen the severity of your diabetes, but probably will be unable to effect a "cure." The required changes are not radical nor overly time-consuming. Rather, they embrace a lifestyle and dietary regimen that physicians recommend for everyone. Although the supportive measures described can not effect a "cure" for Type I diabetics, here too they offer the substantial benefits of better control and improvement in general health. What it boils down to is this: THE DIABETIC PATIENT HIMSELF IS ULTIMATELY RESPONSIBLE FOR LOOKING AFTER HIS DIABETES. His physician and diabetic educator can point the way, but only he can take the necessary steps to do what is required to control his diabetes. Only he can commit to the lifestyle changes required to achieve satisfactory control.

—DONALD A. KULLMAN, M.D.
Editor

WHERE TO FIND HELP

To find a diabetes educator (nurse, registered dietitian, pharmacist, or other professional with experience in diabetes education), call the American Association of Diabetes Educators, toll-free, at 1-800-TEAM-UP-4 (1-800-832-6874). The operator can give you the names of diabetes educators in your zip code.

To find a diabetes education program that has received recognition from the American Diabetes Association, call 1-800-DIABETES (1-800-342-2383). This toll-free call reaches the American Diabetes Association office in your state. Ask for the names and telephone numbers of recognized diabetes education programs near you.

To find a registered dietitian, call toll-free to the Consumer Nutrition Hotline at 1-800-366-1655. This is the National Center for Nutrition and Dietetics of the American Dietetic Association. Ask for the names of registered dietitians in your area who provide diabetes and nutrition counseling.

Acknowledgments

This book covers many aspects of the complex disorder called diabetes mellitus. It is a "How-To" book designed for diabetics to be used under the guidance and approval of their physician. The many clinicians and researchers throughout the years whose published works have contributed to our present understanding of diabetes have made this book possible.

Special thanks are in order for the Eli Lilly Company, Indianapolis, Indiana, who have graciously contributed the material on insulin in Chapter 6 as well as *Guidelines for Healthier Eating With Diabetes*, in Chapter 4. For many years physicians have relied upon Eli Lilly meal plans, of various caloric ranges, to serve as a general guide when utilizing the exchange approach to diabetes dietary management.

I wish to thank the Pritikin Institute for their kind cooperation and permission to use the material incorporated into Chapter 5, *The Pritikin Program and Diabetes*.

Special thanks is also due the Bayer Company, Laboratory Division, Elkhart, Indiana, which has pioneered diagnostic laboratory testing procedures for the home and physician's office. Their generous contribution includes the material utilized in Chapter 11, *Patterns of Control and Sick Day Care*, and Chapter 22, *Straight Talk to Teenagers and Young Adults With Diabetes*.

Acknowledgment is also in order for the U.S. Department of Health and Human Services, National Institute of Health and the Veterans Administration for material dealing with the DCCT, *Long-Term Complications of Diabetes*, *Diabetes in Hispanics*, and *Diabetes in Black Americans*, and material from the V.A. publication *Understanding Diabetes Mellitus*, illustrations by Dawn Potter.

I would like to thank the family of Dr. George F. Schmitt for allowing me to utilize material from his text, *Diabetes for Diabetics*, and also Dr. Ina H. Steinberg, Associate Dean, School of Arts and Sciences, Barry University, for her kind assistance and recommendations.

To all the people at Lifetime Books—Donald Lessne, Brian Feinblum, and Vicki Heil—thank you for your help.

Finally, I would like to thank my editor, Dr. Donald A. Kullman. Dr. Kullman is a graduate of the NYU-Bellevue Hospital Medical Center. He is a widely published medical author known for his ability to explain complicated medical subjects in easy-to-understand language. He has graciously contributed the material for Chapter 16, *Diabetes, Lipids, and Atherosclerosis*.

—SEYMOUR ALTERMAN, M.D., F.A.C.P.

Is a "Cure" for Diabetes Possible?

HOW TO CONTROL DIABETES is filled with current information, based on the most recent scientifically achieved results. This book addresses every significant issue facing today's patients with diabetes. Additionally, Dr. Seymour L. Alterman's book explores cutting-edge research now being performed in laboratories throughout the world, involving the transplantation of islet cell tissues from the pancreas: research that may allow Type I diabetics to eliminate the multiple daily injections of insulin that are required today.

One research group, working with chimpanzees, has transplanted pancreatic tissue, shielded by a protective membrane from the body's normal rejection phenomena. Another group of scientists is working on an attempt to harvest large quantities of the insulin-secreting islet cells from a single donor pancreas. Previously, multiple donors were required to provide a sufficient amount of islet cell tissue. University of Miami researchers are hoping to prevent rejection reactions by mixing transplanted bone marrow cells from the donor with the bone marrow of the recipient. This procedure, if successful, may allow acceptance of the donor islet cells and avoid the marked toxicity associated with current immunosuppressive drugs. Hopefully, this type of painstaking research will result in a cure for diabetes in the not-too-distant future. Until then, Dr. Alterman reminds the reader of currently available knowledge that can ameliorate this disease and reduce the risks of the serious long-term complications of diabetes.

Please refer to our final chapter, *Hope for the Future,* for a more detailed analysis of the latest scientific studies and advancements in the treatment of diabetes.

1

What Is Diabetes Mellitus?

- Metabolic Disorder
- History
- Classifications

Diabetes is a disorder of metabolism—the way our bodies use food for energy, growth, and cellular repair. The most apparent disturbance is with carbohydrate metabolism and is classically characterized by high blood sugar and the excretion of sugar in the urine. To understand diabetes, we must briefly review the normal conversion of food substances into energy by the body. As we walk down the street, hit a baseball, or just take a breath, we expend energy. The body obtains its energy from ingested "fuel" in the form of the food we eat—carbohydrates (sugars and starches), proteins, and fats. Food must be acted upon by digestive enzymes in the stomach and intestinal tract before it can be absorbed. Complex carbohydrates such as those in vegetables and whole grains are composed of long-chain molecules which are broken down by the digestive enzymes to their simple sugar components. All the simple sugars are converted to glucose, the form of sugar required by the cells for physiological functions.

Sugar is absorbed from the intestinal tract into the bloodstream and transported throughout the body, where it is used to provide the energy for daily activities and body metabolism. Any excess is stored away as fat for future use. Each of the billions of cells that make up your body is surrounded by a cell membrane. The sugar must cross that membrane to enter the cell and be utilized. The hormone insulin, manufactured by the pancreas and secreted directly into the bloodstream, plays a vital role in transporting the glucose across the cell membrane. It is the key that opens the cell door to allow the glucose in.

When we eat, the pancreas automatically produces the right amount of insulin to move the glucose from our blood into our cells. In people with diabetes, however, the pancreas either produces little or no insulin, or the body cells are unable to respond to the insulin that is produced. Consequently, glucose builds up in the blood, overflows into the urine, and passes out of the body. Thus, the body loses its main source of fuel even though the blood contains abnormally high levels of glucose. It is an *absolute* or *relative* lack of insulin that defines the disease, diabetes mellitus.

THE HISTORY OF DIABETES MELLITUS

Diabetes is an ancient disorder recognized by its symptoms as early as 400 B.C. It derived its present name in the second century A.D. from a Greek word, meaning "run through a siphon." The Latin word for honey, "mellitus," appeared much later. In 1775, Matthew Dobson, an Englishman, proved through fermentation experiments that the sweet taste in urine of diabetics was actually due to sugar. In 1889, two German scientists, Drs. von Mering and Minkowski, were the first to note that removal of the pancreas, an abdominal organ, from animals caused the syndrome known as diabetes mellitus.

It was shown later that clusters of specialized cells

located in the pancreas actually manufactured, stored, and released a hormone called *insulin* into the blood stream. These cells were given the name "Islets of Langerhans," after their discoverer, Paul Langerhans. These vital "beta" cells act like a tiny thermostat, constantly measuring the blood sugar and releasing just the right amount of insulin to prevent the sugar from going either too high or too low.

In the early years, it was noted that diabetic patients were often obese and developed marked thirst and frequency of urination. As the disease progressed, the patient would try the various nostrums of the day: special diets, fasting, herbal or tribal medicaments, barley water, and even bloodletting. Of course, these therapeutic efforts were to no avail because the real culprit was the absolute or relative absence of the hormone, insulin.

In 1921, a young surgeon, Frederick Banting, with the assistance of Charles H. Best, a medical student who worked in the physiology department at the University of Toronto (and, incidentally, suffered from diabetes himself), made an extract of the tiny pancreatic islet cells and was the first to inject this extract into animals, observing a dramatic fall in blood sugar. Soon, human patients with diabetes were given this "new" insulin treatment, and the modern era in the long and dismal history of diabetes was to begin. Dr. Banting received the Nobel Prize for this important discovery.

Purification and standardization of insulin was undertaken, and prolongation of its action was finally achieved by adding proteins and zinc to the insulin extracted from animals, primarily cows and pigs. Today we use "human" insulin made semisynthetically from pork insulin, or biologically engineered, utilizing complicated recombinant-DNA technology. This has been of great value in reducing the allergic reactions that were sometimes seen with animal insulins.

In later chapters, we shall take an in-depth look at the different types of insulin and their use as well as oral antidiabetic medications.

In summary, diabetes is a chronic metabolic syndrome characterized by high blood sugar, a marked deficiency of insulin, or functionally inadequate insulin, causing, when untreated, deranged metabolism of carbohydrates, fats, and proteins, and leading to chronic long-term complications such as accelerated vascular disease, changes in nerve, kidney, and eye tissue, resulting in organ-specific degenerative processes.

There are two major classifications of *primary* diabetes mellitus: Type I, also known as insulin-dependent diabetes mellitus (IDDM), and Type II, also known as non-insulin-dependent diabetes mellitus (NIDDM). Type I is distinct from Type II in cause, clinical presentation, course, and treatment management. These differences will be discussed in Chapter 2.

Secondary diabetes occurs when there is damage to the pancreas from trauma, tumors, deposits of iron, inflammation of the pancreas (particularly chronic pancreatitus associated with alcoholism), liver disease, medications, and hormonal abnormalities including those that result from the administration of steroids. These causes of diabetes are relatively rare.

Diabetes, not infrequently associated with pregnancy, requires special monitoring. Non-diabetics who develop glucose intolerance during pregnancy have what is called gestational diabetes. The relationship between pregnancy and diabetes is dealt with separately in Chapter 3, *Gestational Diabetes (Diabetes and Pregnancy).*

CRITERIA FOR ESTABLISHING THE DIAGNOSIS OF DIABETES

In the nineteenth century, the diagnosis of diabetes was established by actually tasting and noting the sweetness of the urine. Fortunately, scientific advances have made this crude testing method obsolete. Diabetes is suspected in persons with the classic signs and symptoms of the disorder as well as a high level of glucose in the blood and urine. In asymptomatic individuals, high blood sugar levels alone are usually sufficient to establish the diagnosis. However, it is possible to have some elevation of the blood sugar and even to spill sugar in the urine without having diabetes.

The National Diabetes Data Group (NDDG) has established criteria for diagnosing diabetes by blood testing. In those individuals suspected of having diabetes in whom the fasting blood sugar is less than 140 mg/dl, an oral glucose tolerance test is indicated. This test consists of drinking a solution containing 75 grams of glucose and measuring the blood glucose at prescribed intervals. Normally the blood sugar level rises after the glucose is drunk and then returns to normal.

Normal test results consist of a fasting level less than 115 mg/dl, a peak level less than 200 mg/dl, and a two-hour level less than 140 mg/dl. If the plasma glucose level at two hours is 200 mg/dl or greater and at least one value between zero and two hours is also 200 mg/dl or greater, the diagnosis of diabetes is established. Before a final diagnosis of diabetes is made, however, the test should be repeated and again found to be within the diagnostic range. The NDDG criteria for the diagnosis of diabetes have been set sufficiently high that age adjustment of the criteria is unnecessary.

National Diabetes Data Group Criteria for Interpretation of Oral Glucose Tolerance Test with Use of Venous Plasma or Serum Utilizing a 75 gram Carbohydrate Load*

Fasting or Hours After Glucose Load	Normal	Impaired Glucose Tolerance*	Diabetes**
Fasting	<115	<140	≥140 mg/dl or
1/2 hour and/or 1 hour and/or 1-1/2 hours	<200	≥200	≥200mg/dl
2 hours	<140	140-199	≥200mg/dl

<= less than
>= as much as, or more than
* Values greater than normal, but below criteria for impaired glucose tolerance are designated not diagnostic.
** To establish a diagnosis of diabetes in children a fasting value is required to be ≥ 140 mg/dl in addition to the 1 and 2 hour elevations of the blood glucose.

IMPAIRED GLUCOSE TOLERANCE

Glucose tolerance is said to be impaired when blood glucose levels are higher than normal but not sufficiently high to be diagnostic of diabetes. Those with impaired glucose tolerance may remain unchanged, improve, or eventually go on to develop diabetes.

The following criteria are necessary to qualify for the diagnosis of impaired glucose tolerance according to the standards set by the NDDG: a fasting plasma glucose level less than 140 mg/dl, a two-hour level between 140 and 199 mg/dl, and an intervening value of 200 mg/dl or greater. Although the NDDG criteria make no specific recommendation for age adjustment in evaluating test results, an adjustment may be indicated for the elderly—an allowance of a 10 mg/dl increase for each decade over the age of fifty for the two-hour level may be appropriate.

The term "borderline diabetes" is no longer used to describe those with IGT. The current classification has also eliminated the poorly understood terms "latent diabetes," subclinical, and chemical diabetes and placed them in the IGT category. Likewise, the designation "juvenile diabetes" for Type I and "maturity onset" for Type II are outmoded, misleading, and inaccurate. Age of onset does not necessarily determine the type of diabetes.

AMERICAN DIABETES ASSOCIATION (ADA) RECOMMENDATIONS FOR DIAGNOSING DIABETES

New evidence that diabetes complications may begin at lower blood sugar levels than previously thought have prompted the ADA to change its criteria for diagnosing diabetes. The new recommendations suggest that routine screening be performed on all adults every three years, starting by age forty-five. A fasting plasma glucose level of 126 mg/dl or higher is said to be indicative of diabetes. Fasting levels between 110 and 125 mg/dl are called "impaired fasting glucose." Patients in this category are believed to be at high risk for developing diabetes. The fasting plasma glucose level was chosen because of its convenience and cost effectiveness. Nevertheless, the oral glucose tolerance test remains the gold standard for evaluating diabetes.

2

Type I and Type II Diabetes: Two Different Disorders

- Definitions
- Characteristics
- Ketoacidosis

Type I diabetes, also called insulin-dependent diabetes mellitus (IDDM), was formerly known as juvenile diabetes. Type II diabetes, also called non-insulin-dependent diabetes mellitus (NIDDM), was formerly called maturity-onset diabetes. These two forms of diabetes vary greatly in cause, course, and treatment. Although there are common elements present in both disorders, they represent two significantly different disease complexes.

Type I diabetes is a chronic autoimmune disease that leads to the destruction of all of the insulin-producing beta cells of the pancreas, resulting in an absolute deficiency of insulin. To correct the deficit, people with this form of diabetes must take insulin by injection. Without insulin, they are unable to utilize glucose, causing the body to metabolize fatty acids for energy, a process that leads to a life-threatening metabolic disorder called ketoacidosis.

In Type II diabetes, the beta cells of the pancreas produce insulin, but the body's cells are resistant to its physiological action. Although the pancreas manufactures and secretes insulin, it is unable to secrete enough

8

to overcome that resistance. People with Type II diabetes may be treated with oral hypoglycemic medications (drugs that stimulate insulin production or sensitize the body's cells to insulin's effects). Usually, they do not require insulin to control their disease. There are perhaps as many as seventeen million people in the United States who have diabetes, of whom nine million are unaware of their disease. The explanation for this phenomenon is the great variability of presenting symptoms and the severity of the clinical course that may occur in any given patient.

Type I diabetes often begins abruptly, whereas in Type II (NIDDM) the onset is usually gradual, often remaining asymptomatic for many years. It is not unusual for NIDDM to remain unrecognized for 10–12 years, during which period complications may silently progress. Fifteen to 20% of individuals with undiagnosed diabetes mellitus already have diabetic retinopathy and 5 to 10% already have proteinuria, indicative of kidney disease, when first seen by a physician. Many people are under the mistaken impression that Type II diabetes is not as severe as Type I diabetes. Type II diabetes, if ignored, can cause equally severe health problems, although there may be some variation in the types and patterns of the medical problems encountered.

In Type I diabetes, the onset of elevated blood sugar usually begins before age 30, with a peak incidence between 12–14. Its former name, juvenile diabetes, refers to a disease complex most commonly seen in the young, although it may also occur in older age groups. Increased thirst, hunger, and frequency of urination, particularly at night, associated with unexplained weight loss, fatigue, and apathy, in spite of increased appetite, herald the onset of Type I diabetes in its classical form.

Occasionally, a severe cold or other viral infection will lead to one of the major complications of Type I diabetes, acute ketoacidosis. This metabolic disorder, a grave, life-threatening complication, must be treated rapidly and with expertise by a physician well versed in caring for this condition. Ketoacidosis will be explored in greater detail later in this chapter.

In the early stage of his disease, the Type I diabetic patient may have periods of remission for varying lengths of time, but the disorder returns and eventually becomes constant. Type I (IDDM) is usually treated with two divided doses of insulin daily and requires careful attention to diet and exercise in order to maintain adequate control. Researchers believe IDDM is caused by a combination of factors, with genetics and environmental stress, including exposure to common viruses and other substances early in life, playing major roles. In other words, there is a genetic predisposition conferred by a "diabetic" gene or genes. Genetic factors are clearly important in the cause and susceptibility of diabetes. This has been verified by studies of both identical and nonidentical twins. But it is also clear that while genetic factors are important in both NIDDM and IDDM, *they are only predisposing components* and must interact with environmental influences to produce diabetes in a given individual.

IDDM affects only about 10% to 15% of the entire diabetic population. Unable to produce insulin, sugar is not able to enter cells and be available to be used for energy.

The proper management of IDDM—with careful attention to administration of insulin, checking blood sugars, proper diet and exercise, and working with a physician and diabetic educator—is the mainstay of treatment and will be dealt with in later chapters.

With modern knowledge and treatment, there is no longer a need for fear, anger, and confusion to weigh heavily on the young diabetic. By following simple rules, as outlined in this book, many of the false myths and anecdotal horror stories about diabetes will be laid to rest and a bright, new outlook on life will take its place.

Type II diabetes, or NIDDM, differs sharply from Type I in many important respects. The onset is usually insidious rather than precipitous and is far more common after age 40, reaching a peak incidence between 60–65. Type II patients make up 85% to 90% of the total diabetic population in the United States. Approximately 80% of Type II patients are obese and may have few or no symptoms. Blood glucose levels in NIDDM do not usually rise or fall rapidly as in IDDM, and ketoacidosis is quite rare. Blood levels of insulin in NIDDM may be normal or even increased. This continued ability of the pancreas to manufacture insulin facilitates treatment. More women than men develop NIDDM.

There is no simple explanation for the causes of Type II diabetes. While eating sugar, for example, does not cause diabetes, eating large amounts of sugar and other rich, fatty foods can cause weight gain. Most people who develop Type II diabetes are overweight, but scientists do not fully understand why obesity increases someone's chances of developing diabetes. Current research suggests obesity increases insulin resistance. This would help explain why obesity is such an important risk factor.

A major cause of Type II diabetes is insulin resistance. Scientists are still searching for the cause of insulin resistance, but they have identified two possibilities. The first points to a defect in the insulin receptors on cells. Like an appliance that must be plugged into an electrical outlet, insulin needs to bind to a cell receptor to function. Several things can go wrong with the receptor mechanism. There may be too few receptors for insulin to bind to, or there may be a defect in the receptors that prevents the insulin from binding.

A second possible factor may be a defect in the process that occurs after insulin plugs into the receptor. Insulin may successfully bind to the receptors, but the cells do not read the signal to metabolize the glucose. Research is currently seeking to determine why this might happen.

While antibodies that destroy the islet cells of the pancreas are found commonly in IDDM, the incidence is less than 3% in NIDDM. It is important to understand that although the pancreas is able to store and secrete insulin in Type II diabetes, the overall pattern of its response to the ingestion of carbohydrate is delayed. Some of Type II diabetics will eventually require insulin treatment; most however will respond to weight loss, exercise, diet, and if necessary, oral medications.

We now know there are strong genetic determinants for obesity and insulin resistance. There are definite racial and ethnic differences in the incidence of NIDDM, with a very high rate, for example, among Pima Native Americans in Arizona, Hispanics, and African Americans. Environmental factors as well as genetic factors undoubtedly contribute to the increased incidence in these ethnic groups. Studies have shown that when excessive obesity is factored out, the incidence of diabetes is no greater for African Americans than for Caucasians. At the present time, we can only state categorically that susceptibility to contract NIDDM can be found in the genome at conception. The body cell, be it a muscle, fat, or other cell, does not respond appropriately to the insulin that is present, and the blood sugar rises. It is this sustained rise in blood sugar, above normal through the years, that is responsible for the later long-term complications of diabetes.

KETOACIDOSIS: A CRUCIAL COMPLICATION

Though rare, ketoacidosis is an important, at times life-threatening, acute complication of diabetes that must be promptly recognized and appropriately treated.

As noted, the lack of insulin in the blood results in an inability of the muscle, liver, and fat cells to "take in" the sugar and convert it into energy for vital life processes. Even though the blood sugar is rising, the cells are unable to obtain their fuel. When this happens, storage depots in the liver release stored glucose, and the blood sugar rises even higher as the body attempts to correct the lack of glucose at the cellular level. Without treatment, the excessive sugar in the blood is excreted in the urine, carrying with it large quantities of water, causing dehydration. The body now turns to stored fat to provide the energy it needs to function, and it is this "lipolysis" (abnormal fat metabolism) that causes a problem. As the fats are broken down, they are converted into waste products called ketones and free fatty acids (incomplete breakdown products of fat metabolism); hence, the term *ketoacidosis*. Ketones spill into the urine and are easily detected by a simple laboratory test. Some ketones are also excreted by the lungs, giving rise to the unique, fruity acetone breath associated with ketoacidosis. If the blood ketone level rises too high, life-threatening ketoacidosis can develop. It is not necessary to understand the biochemical changes of ketoacidosis in order to recognize the signs and symptoms that will alert you to seek prompt treatment for this condition.

Whenever two consecutive blood sugars are above 200 mg/dl in Type I diabetes, the urine must be tested for ketones. Although Type II diabetics are not ketosis prone, whenever they are subject to stress from infections or illness, they too should check their urine for ketones.

Signs and Symptoms of Ketoacidosis

Increased thirst and urination
Dehydration
Blurred vision
Acetone breath
Weight loss
Abdominal pain
Ketones in the urine
Blood sugar usually over 200 mg/dl
Nausea, vomiting
Rapid pulse, and often labored breathing
Lethargy

TREATMENT OF KETOACIDOSIS

When symptoms suggestive of ketoacidosis appear, it is important to check blood sugar levels. If a high blood sugar level is found and ketones are present in the urine, a dose of regular, fast-acting, insulin is indicated. Often an extra dose of regular insulin and exercise can prevent ketoacidosis from progressing to the stage where hospitalization becomes necessary. In any case, treatment of ketoacidosis should be handled by your physician, but in an emergency, you should be taken to the nearest hospital with trained emergency room physicians. The basic treatment consists of providing adequate insulin to reverse the metabolic defects and to correct the deficit of body fluids and electrolytes. The electrolytes are charged minerals that play important roles in physiological functions. A few of the more important ones are potassium, sodium, and chloride that maintain the body's delicate fluid balance. The bicarbonate ion is responsible for keeping the acid base balance of the blood (the Ph) within the narrow range compatible with life. Electrolytes are lost whenever there is excessive fluid loss as a result of fever, diarrhea, or vomiting. The exact amount of insulin, saline, and other electrolytes required to restore physiological harmony must be carefully monitored by the treating physician and ancillary personnel, but almost invariably, the patient will respond favorably and return to the pre-acidotic state within a relatively short time, feeling much better.

HYPEROSMOLAR NONKETOTIC SYNDROME (HNKS)

The Hyperosmolar Nonketotic Syndrome consists of the association of an extremely high blood sugar, 800mg/dl or higher, mental aberrations ranging from disorientation and confusion to coma, in the absence of ketones in the urine, generally occuring in Type II diabetics. (Note: HNKS also occurs in nondiabetics, in association with such medical conditions as Cushing's Syndrome, acromegaly, pancreatitis, certain drugs, severe burns, heat stroke, etc.)

HNKS resembles diabetic ketoacidosis, but since insulin is available in the Type II diabetic, the derangement in fat metabolism that causes the incomplete burning of the fats with the formation of ketone bodies does not occur. In other words, even though the insulin cannot work properly in Type II diabetes, fat metabolism is not markedly deranged. The cause of coma in both cases, however, is the same. The body attempts to lower the elevated blood sugar by excreting the excess sugar in the urine. This results in water loss and dehydration, which explains the excessive thirst and urination. Although the blood does not become acidotic in HNKS as in keto-acidosis, it does become more concentrated as the blood volume decreases with the loss of fluid in the urine. The term "hyperosmolar" means literally "increased concentration" (of the blood). The symptoms of HNKS are similar to those of diabetic ketoacidosis: thirst, frequent urination, nausea, labored breathing, dry skin, mental confusion, and drowsiness progressing to coma. Prevention of this serious condition is another reason why home monitoring of blood glucose plays such an important role in diabetes management. Persistent elevation of blood glucose above 400 mg/dl for 12 hours, despite additional insulin, requires immediate medical attention. Once significant dehydration has occurred, hospitalization is mandatory to correct the fluid and electrolyte balance.

CHARACTERISTIC FEATURES OF THE TWO MAJOR TYPES OF PRIMARY DIABETES MELLITUS

	Type I or Insulin-Dependent <u>Diabetes Mellitus:</u>	Type II or Non-Insulin-Dependent <u>Diabetes Mellitus:</u>
	Juvenile-onset diabetes mellitus; Ketosis-prone diabetes mellitus; Insulin-deficient diabetes mellitus	Maturity-onset diabetes mellitus; Ketosis-resistant diabetes mellitus; Insulin-resistant diabetes mellitus

Clinical Features

Age of Onset	Usually before age 30; peak incidence at age 12–14	Usually after age 40; peak incidence at age 60–65

Clinical Onset	Usually abrupt, may be gradual	Usually insidious
Symptoms	Polyuria, polydipsia, polyphagia, weight loss, acidosis	Often asymptomatic; may have fatigue, weakness, infections
Nutritional Status	Usually normal	Obesity in 80–90%
Ketosis-Proneness	Frequent, especially if treatment insufficient	Uncommon except during infection or unusual stress
Carbohydrate-Intolerance	Marked	Mild, moderate, or marked
Remission Phase	Often occurs	Following weight reduction
Stability	Labile, wide fluctuations in blood glucose common	Relatively stable, blood glucose fluctuations less marked
Insulin Responsiveness	Sensitive	Usually resistant
Control of Diabetes	Often difficult	Usually not difficult

Epidemiology

	Insulin-Dependent	*Non-Insulin-Dependent*
Proportion of	Less than 10%	Greater than 90%
Sex Predilection	About equal distribution	Female preponderance
Concordance in Identical Twins	Less than 50%	Greater than 90%
Islet Cell Antibodies	40–80% at onset	Less than 5%
Association with Autoimmune Disorders	Not uncommon	Rare

Endogenous Insulin

	"Low-output"	"High-output"
Pancreatic	Very low	Normal, slightly diminished, or increased
Fasting Plasma	Absent or low	Normal or elevated
Response to Glucose	None to negligible	(1) Adequate—even elevated—but delayed or (2) Diminished but not absent

Pathology

Islet Mass	Markedly diminished	Minimally altered
B-cell Mass	Markedly diminished	Variable—may be slightly decreased or hypertropic

Therapeutic Requirements

	Insulin-Dependent	*Non-Insulin-Dependent*
Diet	Mandatory to balance food intake with energy expenditure and insulin dosage	Diet alone may be adequate for therapy; clinical remission may follow weight reduction
Insulin	Necessary for all patients; most patients require at least two doses daily	Necessary for 20–30% of patients; single, daily dose often adequate
Oral Agents (Sulfonylureas, Metformin, etc.)	Not efficacious	Frequently efficacious
Physical Activity	Must be balanced with food intake and insulin	May improve insulin action

3

Gestational Diabetes
(Diabetes and Pregnancy)

- Incidence
- Diagnosis
- Management and Prognosis

In the past, pregnancy for women with diabetes posed a major threat to both the mother and the fetus. Today, the prognosis has changed, due to more intensive control of diabetes *before* conception and meticulous management throughout the pregnancy.

Many studies have shown that achieving excellent control of blood sugar before and during pregnancy reduces maternal complications to about the same rate as the general population. It also substantially reduces infant mortality and complications.

Tight control *before* getting pregnant and during the first three months of pregnancy is especially important since the first trimester is the period of formation of the major fetal organs and therefore the time when the developing fetus is most vulnerable to damage from elevated blood sugars. Poorly controlled diabetes may lead to fetal malformations, intrauterine death, and a higher rate of miscarriage. Pregnancy has an effect on insulin dosage during the gestational period. Often, less insulin is needed in the first trimester; insulin requirements then rise until term and delivery.

Women who have had no previous signs or laboratory indication of diabetes prior to the pregnancy, but who develop abnormally high levels of glucose during pregnancy, have gestational diabetes mellitus (GDM). In other words, the designation GDM is restricted to patients whose glucose intolerance develops during pregnancy. Many of these patients, as well as many of those who have mild Type II diabetes, probably do not require as "tight" or intensive management as does the pregnant Type I diabetic unless the diabetic status deteriorates during the pregnancy. Monitoring of glucose and careful evaluation of glycohemoglobin levels (a special blood test that serves as a barometer of long-term control) are important throughout pregnancy.

GDM occurs in about 2% to 3% of all pregnancies and is more apt to occur in women who are over thirty, overweight, and/or have a family history of diabetes. Previous delivery of a large baby (nine pounds or more) increases the need for close surveillance of the blood sugar level by the doctor. GDM is more common in Hispanic Americans, African Americans, and Native Americans. GDM develops most frequently between the 24th and 28th weeks of pregnancy and usually goes away after the baby is born.

Because diabetes can have serious consequences for the fetus as well as the mother, it is now routine for obstetricians to test for GDM as soon as the diagnosis of pregnancy is made.

A blood test is the only way to make the diagnosis of GDM. If you have had GDM during an earlier pregnancy, your doctor will monitor your blood sugar closely. If you have never had GDM, following your prenatal evaluation, you will be screened again between the 24th and 28th weeks of pregnancy. This screening test consists of drinking a sugar beverage containing a known quantity of glucose followed by a blood glucose test one hour later. You can eat normally before this test. If the test shows elevation of the blood sugar, you will be asked to take a 3-hour glucose tolerance test (GTT). It is important that you do not eat or drink on the morning of your GTT. This test will give a definitive answer to whether or not you have GDM.

The normal upper limit of *fasting* plasma glucose in pregnancy is 105 mg/dl. To diagnose GDM, two or more of the blood sugar levels after a 100-gram oral glucose load must meet or exceed the following values:

Sample 1—Fasting	105 mg/dl
Sample 2—1 Hour	190 mg/dl
Sample 3—2 Hour	165 mg/dl
Sample 4—3 Hour	145 mg/dl

When patients exceed these levels, especially when confirmed by a repeated test, a diagnosis of GDM can be made by the obstetrician. As noted, if the initial blood sugar test is within the normal range, obstetricians will routinely repeat a fasting sugar at intervals during the pregnancy.

The fasting glucose level is lower during pregnancy because of the constant transfer of glucose to the fetus as the mother supplies nourishment via the placenta. Additionally, many metabolic and hormonal changes occur in pregnancy that act physiologically to antagonize the action of insulin, creating a form of insulin "resistance." This phenomenon has the effect of raising blood sugar levels and making rigorous control of diabetes during pregnancy even more difficult.

Another serious complication of poorly controlled blood sugars in pregnancy is the possible development of ketoacidosis. Ketones are particularly hazardous to the fetus and ketoacidosis is associated with a marked increase in fetal mortality. Therefore, checking the mother's urine for ketones is a necessity throughout pregnancy. Ketones in the urine may be due to a patient missing a meal or snack and the body relying on the breakdown of stored fat for nutrition, at least on a temporary basis. Increasing the caloric intake or taking more frequent snacks will correct this "ketonuria." Eating a snack before bedtime to protect against ketone formation during the night is recommended by some obstetricians.

When maternal blood glucose rises, it passes through the placenta into the baby's bloodstream. Because insulin cannot penetrate the placenta, the fetus's blood sugar levels are abnormally high when the mother's diabetes is out of control. The chronically elevated blood sugar supplies extra calories that cause excessive fetal weight gain. The large size of the fetus often leads to premature birth, or, in some cases, necessitates a Caesarian section to facilitate delivery. Furthermore, the baby's own pancreas may have become accustomed to making extra insulin to handle the increased sugar load. The baby's pancreas may then continue to manufacture extra insulin after birth, when it is no longer needed, causing low blood sugar or hypoglycemia. This is most likely to happen when the blood sugars are high during the last few days of pregnancy.

For reasons already noted, if a person has been diagnosed with diabetes *before* the onset of pregnancy, intensification of diabetic control and careful attention to diet, exercise, and insulin requirements become essential and urgent. Therefore, frequent glucose monitoring with fingerstick blood sugars must be done on a regimen advised by the physician or diabetic educator. This usually requires determination of blood sugars before and sometimes after meals, before and sometimes after exercise, and whenever symptoms of excessive fatigue or illness occur.

Remember, oral hypoglycemic drugs should not be taken by the diabetic mother because of possible adverse effects on the fetus.

With the emphasis on careful dietary control, home-glucose monitoring, physician-recommended exercise, and intensive diabetic control, the vast majority of diabetic pregnancies result in normal, healthy newborn babies.

The blood sugar of most patients with GDM will return to normal after delivery. However, the diabetes does persist in about 2% of all women who have GDM. Another 8% have blood sugars that are higher than normal, but not high enough to be called diabetes—a condition called *impaired glucose tolerance*. Up to 60% of women who have had GDM will get diabetes later in life and should be checked at 6-month intervals. Obese women have the greatest risk of developing lifelong diabetes. Of those patients who maintain normal weight after pregnancy, less than 25% will eventually develop diabetes.

All patients who have elevated blood sugars during their pregnancy should have blood sugar evaluations after delivery at intervals determined by their physician.

A slightly yellow skin color (jaundice) frequently occurs in newborns. It is caused by a body chemical called bilirubin. Usually this is transient and resolves spontaneously without treatment. Jaundice is more likely to be severe in babies whose mothers develop gestational diabetes. A simple light treatment is usually all that is required to help absorb the extra buildup of bilirubin, the blood breakdown product that causes the changes in skin color.

The management of the pregnant woman with known previous diabetes and the pregnant woman who develops diabetes during pregnancy (GDM) is the same. Adherence to a well-balanced meal plan (adjusted for insulin requirements), maintenance of prescribed blood glucose levels, and regular exercise is essential.

It is important to include all of the basic food groups in the meal plan. Total pregnancy weight gain should not exceed 25 to 35 pounds. Caffeine, alcohol, concentrated sweets, and artificial sweeteners are to be avoided. Blood sugars should be tested before breakfast, one hour after breakfast, one hour after lunch, and one hour after dinner. Your doctor may prescribe a different schedule for checking the blood sugars for your individual case.

In pregnant Type I diabetics, the physician will not want the glucose to exceed 170–180 mg/dl. In gestational diabetes, the goal is to keep the fasting sugar below 105 mg /dl.

The optimal time for delivery depends on fetal status and maturity. The goal is to allow the pregnancy to go at least 35 weeks and then check the patient carefully until the 37th or 38th week.

The urine should be routinely checked for ketones, remembering the previous admonitions. It is best to check the urine for ketones in the morning before eating.

Exercise is particularly important in GDM. Twenty- to thirty-minute walks after meals can help utilize excess blood sugar. It is best to let your doctor determine the correct amount of exercise during your pregnancy.

A glucose tolerance test 6 weeks after delivery, and then at least once a year, is recommended for follow-up care. With modern management, pregnant women who have had either a previous diagnosis of diabetes or gestational diabetes, can now, with appropriate education, proper meal planning, careful control of blood sugar throughout pregnancy, adequate exercise, and proper motivation, look forward to a happy and healthy life for themselves as well as their newborn babies.

4

Guidelines for Healthier Eating With Diabetes*

- Importance for Diabetic Control
- Exchange Lists
- Meal Planning

Eating healthy foods is one of the most basic and important tools of diabetes management. The right foods can help control blood sugar and protect long-term health. Every person with diabetes should have a personal meal plan developed by a registered dietitian (RD) or other qualified professional. This preplanned menu sheet is a good start. Use it to begin to learn about diabetes meal planning and to guide your choices until you can get a personalized plan to meet your long-term needs.

What You Need to Do

- Realize that the best food choices to control diabetes are healthy choices for the whole family.
- Reach and stay at a desirable body weight. Extra body fat makes it harder to control blood sugar.
- Eat a variety of foods—"well-balanced meals"—at regular times each day to balance diabetes medicines and control hunger.

*Material in this chapter courtesy Eli Lilly and Company, Indianapolis, Indiana.

- Be physically active. Do an activity or exercise you enjoy at least 3 or 4 times a week and look for ways to put more activity in your daily routine.
- See your health care team regularly to check your diabetes. Your doctor, dietitian, diabetes educator, and pharmacist can make the job of staying healthy much easier.

EASY STEPS TO HEALTHIER EATING

Eat Less Fat, Especially Animal Fat

- Eat fewer high-fat foods like cold cuts, sausage, and nuts. Cut down on add-ons such as butter, margarine, lard, oil, shortening, salad dressing, and gravy.
- Eat less fried food. Try baking, broiling, steaming, grilling, and poaching instead.
- Reduce your use of high-fat cuts of red meat. Instead, have chicken and turkey (without skin), fish, lean meats, and vegetarian dishes such as beans.
- Choose low-fat and skim dairy products. Avoid whole milk, cream, high-fat cheeses, and eggs.
- Season food with low-fat flavorings. Try lemon or lime juice, flavored vinegars, low-calorie salad dressings, low-fat yogurt, or small amounts of wine instead of butter, margarine, sour cream, and other high-fat choices.

Eat More Starches and Foods High in Fiber

- Eat starches—like potatoes, pasta, grains, and vegetables—and fresh fruit every day. Choose whole-grain breads, cereals, and crackers.

• Regularly include peas, beans, rice, bran, and oats in your food choices.

Eat Less Sugar

• Drink low-calorie, sugar-free soda instead of the regularly sweetened type.
• Eat less table sugar, honey, jelly, candy, cookies, cake, pie, and other sweets.
• Find a sugar substitute you like and use it instead of table sugar. Look for prepared foods made with sugar substitutes instead of real sugar.
• When you want something sweet, try diet gelatin (with or without fruit), graham crackers, angel food cake, artificially sweetened nonfat yogurt, or low-sugar jams and jellies.

Use Less Salt

• Keep the salt shaker off the table. Keep pepper, onion and garlic powders, and other low-salt seasonings handy instead.
• Cook without adding salt. Flavor foods with spices and herbs instead.
• Eat less salty food. Canned soups, pickles, hot dogs, bacon, sausage, snack chips, and convenience and fast foods often contain large amounts of salt.

HOW TO PLAN MEALS FOR BETTER DIABETES CONTROL

The 1,200–2,000 calorie charts in the next section show a method of planning meals that works well for people who have diabetes. In it, similar foods are divided into groups called "exchange lists."* An exchange meal plan shows a certain number of servings from each group to be eaten every day. Foods on the same list can be substituted for each other in the serving sizes shown. For example, List 4 shows you that 1 small apple is equal to 1 1/4 cups of fresh strawberries. This information makes it possible to eat many different kinds of foods while still making good choices for diabetes control.

For example, when your meal plan calls for 1 starch/bread exchange at a meal, you can select any food from List 1 in the amount shown: 1 slice of bread, half of an English muffin, or 1 corn tortilla, for example. If your plan calls for 2 or more servings from a group at 1 meal, you can either increase the serving size of 1 food (2 slices of bread or a whole English muffin, for example) or choose 2 items from the list (1 dinner roll *and* 1/2 cup of mashed potatoes, for example).

The foods in the exchange lists are marked to help you eat more fiber and less salt and cholesterol for better health.

🍀 shows foods that are good sources of fiber.

🖐 shows foods that are high in salt.

🔥 shows foods that are high in cholesterol.

The daily meal plan that follows is an example of how you can plan your meals using the exchange lists. When you plan your own meals, pick foods from the exchange

* *These exchange lists are based on a meal planning system designed by a committee of the American Diabetes and the American Dietetic Association. Eli Lilly and Company gratefully acknowledge the assistance of Diabetes Care and Education, a group of the American Dietetic Association, in developing this revised meal planning tool.*

lists that you enjoy and eat regularly. Eating the right number of servings from each exchange list will help you balance the right amounts of the foods you prefer. This is a big step toward good diabetes control.

Measuring Foods—

Serving size is important. Notice that the sample menu includes the right serving sizes for the meal plan shown. To get the serving size right, measure all foods using standard measuring cups and spoons or a food scale.

All measures are level (not rounded or heaping). Four ounces of raw meat with bone will shrink to 3 ounces after cooking. Use this general rule to estimate your serving of meat from its size before cooking. Other cooked foods should be measured after cooking.

Food Preparation and Selection—

Try preparing old favorites in new ways to meet your healthier eating goals. Stir-frying and steaming are two low-fat cooking methods you can try. Meats can be baked, broiled, roasted, or grilled. Pan-broiling is a low-fat method when a nonstick pan or vegetable oil spray is used instead of butter, margarine, or shortening.

Note—

Everyone with diabetes should have his own individually designed meal plan.

FOOD EXCHANGE LISTS

LIST 1—STARCHES/BREADS

(15 grams carbohydrate, 3 grams protein, a trace of fat, and 80 calories per serving)

Breads, starchy vegetables, and other starchy foods are the cornerstone of every healthy eating plan. Most of their calories come from carbohydrates, which are good sources of energy. Many choices from this group also provide needed fiber, vitamins, and minerals. For better health, prepare and eat these foods with as little added fat as possible, using less butter, margarine, shortening, and oil.

Use the following guide to estimate servings of any plain starch or bread not listed.
- Starchy vegetables, grains, pasta . . . . $^1/_2$ cup
- Breads and cereals . . . . 1 oz

Cereals/Grains/Pasta/ Starchy Vegetables	*Serving Size*
Cereal, cooked (oatmeal, oat bran, cream of wheat, rice, etc.)	$^1/_2$ cup
Dry cereal, any type containing less than 100 calories per 1-oz serving. . . . . (Serving sizes may vary; check box.)	1 oz
Macaroni, noodles, spaghetti, and other pasta, cooked	$^1/_2$ cup
Rice, brown, white, cooked	$^1/_3$ cup
Bulgur, barley, other grains	$^1/_2$ cup
Dried beans, peas, lentils, cooked	$^1/_3$ cup
Lima beans, cooked	$^1/_2$ cup
Corn	$^1/_2$ cup
Corn on the cob (6" piece)	1
Peas, green, cooked	$^1/_2$ cup
Potato, baked, boiled, steamed.	1 small (3 oz)

Potato, mashed with
    nothing added . . . . ¹/₂ cup
Squash, winter, acorn, hubbard . . . . ³/₄ cup
Yam, sweet potato . . . . ¹/₃ cup

Breads
Breads, whole wheat, 🔖 rye, white,
    pumpernickel, raisin, other . . . . 1 slice (1 oz)
Bagel, plain, small . . . . ¹/₂ (1 oz)
Bun, hamburger, hot dog . . . . ¹/₂ (1 oz)
Dinner roll. . . . . 1 small
Sandwich roll, kaiser . . . . ¹/₂ small
English muffin . . . . ¹/₂
Pita pocket (6–8" across) . . . . ¹/₂
Pita pocket (4" across) 1
Tortilla, flour, corn 1

Crackers/Snacks
Animal crackers 8
Graham crackers (2 ¹/₂" square) 3
Melba toast, oblongs 5
Melba toast, rounds 7
Whole wheat or rye crackers
    (80 calories/serving) 4–6
Saltines, unsalted tops 6
Pretzels . . . . ³/₄ oz
Popcorn, plain, popped . . . . 3 cups
Sherbet, any flavor . . . . ¹/₄ cup
Yogurt, frozen, fruit flavor . . . . ¹/₃ cup

Starches/Breads With Fat
(15 grams carbohydrate, 3 grams protein, 5 or more grams
fat, and 125–150 calories per serving)
Count as 1 Starch/Bread serving *and* 1 Fat serving.

Biscuit (2 ½")............................... 1
Cornbread (2" cube)......................... 1
Crackers, butter type........................ 6
French fries (2–3 ½" long)................... 10
🔖 Potato chips.............................. 10
Muffin, small, plain (2–3")................... ½
Taco shell (6") 2

LIST 2—MEAT AND MEAT SUBSTITUTES

Small servings of meat and meat substitutes provide ample protein for daily needs. For better health, choose lean meats, fish, and poultry more often than medium- and high-fat meats and cheeses.

Lean Meats
(7 grams protein, 3 grams fat, and 55 calories per serving)
                                          Serving Size
Chicken or turkey, skin removed................ 1 oz
Lean cuts of beef
   (round, extra lean
   ground round, flank steak, etc.).............. 1 oz
Lean cuts of pork
   (🔖 Canadian bacon, 🔖 ham, etc.)............ 1 oz
Veal (lean chops and roasts) .... 1 oz
Fish, fresh or frozen.......................... 1 oz
Shellfish (clams, crab, lobster,
   scallops, 🔖 shrimp) .... 2 oz
🔖 Tuna, canned in water .... ¼ cup
Cottage cheese, low-fat .... ¼ cup
Egg substitute................................ ¼ cup

Medium-fat Meats
(7 grams protein, 5 grams fat, and 75 calories per serving)
Beef, pork, lamb (most cuts) .... 1 oz

Veal cutlet, ground or cubed,
   unbreaded . . . . 1 oz
🔥 Liver . . . . 1 oz
🔥 Egg 1
Cheese, low-fat, part skim. . . . . 1 oz

High-fat Meats

(7 grams protein, 8 grams fat, and 100 calories per serving)
🔥 Prime beef, 🔥 corned beef . . . . 1 oz
🔥 Spareribs. . . . . 1 oz
🔆 🔥 Sausage, 🔆 🔥 luncheon meat . . . . 1 oz
🔆 🔥 Hot dog. . . . . 1 oz
🔆 🔥 Regular cheese . . . . 1 oz
Peanut butter . . . . 1 Tbsp

LIST 3—VEGETABLES

(5 grams carbohydrate, 2 grams protein, and 25 calories per serving)
Vegetables are a very good source of vitamins and minerals. Many choices from this group also provide some fiber. A serving is ¹/₂ cup of cooked vegetables, ¹/₂ cup of vegetable juice, or 1 cup of raw vegetables. (Starchy vegetables like potatoes, corn, and peas appear on List 1—Starches/Breads. Vegetables that have fewer than 20 calories per serving appear on List 7—Free Foods.)

Asparagus	Cabbage
Beans, green, wax, Italian	Carrots
	Cauliflower
Bean sprouts	Eggplant
Beets	Green onion
Broccoli	Greens, collard,
Brussels sprouts	mustard, etc.

Mushrooms
Okra
Onion
Pea pods (snow peas)
Peppers, red, green,
  yellow
🖎 Sauerkraut
Spinach

Squash, summer,
  crookneck, zucchini
Tomato
🖎 Tomato or vegetable
  juice
Turnip
Water chestnuts

LIST 4—FRUITS

(15 grams carbohydrate and 60 calories per serving)
Fruits provide important vitamins and minerals and are a good source of fiber. To obtain the most fiber from fruits, eat the edible peelings, too, such as those of apples, apricots, and pears.

Use the following guide to estimate servings of any fruit not listed.
- Fresh, canned, or frozen
  fruit, no sugar added . . . . ¹/₂ cup
- Dried fruit . . . . ¹/₄ cup

	Serving Size
Apple, raw (2")	1
Applesauce, no sugar added	¹/₂ cup
Apricot, raw (medium)	4
Banana (9" long)	¹/₂
🖎 Blackberries or 🖎 blueberries, raw	³/₄ cup
Cantaloupe or honeydew melon	1 cup
Cherries, raw (large)	12
Fig, raw (2" across)	2
Grapefruit (medium)	¹/₂
Grapes (small)	15
Kiwi (large)	1

Mandarin oranges. . . . . ³/₄ cup
🌿 Nectarine (2 ¹/₂" across) 1
Orange (2 ¹/₂" across) 1
Papaya . . . . 1 cup
Peach (2 ³/₄" across). . . . . 1 whole or ³/₄ cup
Pear . . . . ¹/₂ large or 1 small
Pineapple, fresh . . . . ³/₄ cup
Plum, raw (2" across) 2
🌿 Strawberries, raw (whole) . . . . 1 ¹/₄ cup
Tangerine (2 ¹/₂" across) 2
Watermelon . . . . 1 ¹/₄ cup

Dried Fruit
🌿 Apricots . . . . 7 halves
🌿 Prunes (medium). 3
Raisins . . . . 2 Tbsp

Fruit Juices
Apple, orange, grapefruit . . . . ¹/₂ cup
Cranberry, grape, prune . . . . ¹/₃ cup

LIST 5—MILK AND MILK PRODUCTS

Milk and milk products are needed throughout life. Choose 2 or more servings a day. Milk products supply calcium and other minerals, vitamins, protein, and carbohydrate. Choose low-fat and skim varieties for better health since these choices have less fat, calories, and cholesterol than whole milk products.

Skim Milk and Skim Milk Products
(12 grams carbohydrate, 8 grams protein, 1 gram fat, and
90–110 calories per serving)

Serving Size

Skim, 1/2%, 1% milk . . . . 8 oz
Buttermilk, low-fat . . . . 8 oz
Evaporated skim milk . . . . 4 oz
Nonfat dry milk powder . . . . 2 2/3 oz (1/3 cup)
Yogurt, nonfat, plain . . . . 8 oz
Yogurt, nonfat, fruited,
    artificially sweetened. . . . . 8 oz
Hot cocoa, artificially sweetened . . . . 1 envelope

Low-fat Milk and Low-fat Milk Products
(12 grams carbohydrate, 8 grams protein, 3 or more
grams fat, and 120–150 calories per serving)
2% milk . . . . 8 oz
Yogurt, low-fat, plain. . . . . 8 oz

Whole Milk and Whole Milk Products
(12 grams carbohydrate, 8 grams protein, 5 or more
grams fat, and 150–170 calories per serving)
*To reduce your intake of cholesterol and saturated fat,
limit or avoid foods in this group.*
Whole milk . . . . 8 oz
Evaporated whole milk . . . . 4 oz
Yogurt, regular, plain. . . . . 8 oz

LIST 6—FATS

(5 grams fat and 45 calories per serving)
*Fats add flavor and moisture to foods but provide few
additional nutrients, such as vitamins and minerals. Note
that serving sizes of fats are small. Choose unsaturated
fats instead of saturated fats to help lower blood cholesterol levels.*

Unsaturated Fats   *Serving Size*

Margarine, stick . . . . 1 tsp

Margarine, tub. . . . . 1 tsp

Margarine, diet . . . . 1 Tbsp

Mayonnaise, regular . . . . 1 tsp

Mayonnaise, reduced-calorie. . . . . 1 Tbsp

Salad dressing, regular . . . . 1 Tbsp

Salad dressing, reduced-calorie . . . . 2 Tbsp

Oil, corn, cottonseed, soybean,
   olive, sunflower, safflower, peanut . . . . 1 tsp

Nuts and seeds. . . . . 1 Tbsp

Saturated Fats

Bacon . . . . 1 slice

Butter . . . . 1 tsp

Nondairy creamer, liquid. . . . . 2 Tbsp

Nondairy creamer, powdered . . . . 4 tsp

Cream, light, table, coffee, sour . . . . 2 Tbsp

Cream, heavy, whipping. 1 Tbsp

Cream cheese. . . . . 1 Tbsp

LIST 7—FREE FOODS

Each free food or drink contains fewer than 20 calories per serving. You may eat as much as you want of free foods that have no serving size listed; you may eat 2 or 3 servings per day of free foods that have serving sizes listed. For better blood sugar control, spread your servings of these extra foods throughout the day.

Drinks

Bouillon or broth,
   no fat

Cocoa powder,
   unsweetened baking
   type (1 Tbsp)

Coffee or tea

Soft drinks, calorie-free,
   including carbonated
   drinks

Fruits
Cranberries or rhubarb,
   no sugar added
   ($^1/_2$ cup)

Condiments
Catsup (1 Tbsp)
🔖 Dill pickles,
   unsweetened
Horseradish
Hot sauce
Mustard
Salad dressing, nonfat,
   low-caloric, including
   mayonnaise-type
   (2 Tbsp)
Taco sauce (2 Tbsp)
Vinegar

Vegetables
Celery
Cucumber
Peppers, hot
Radishes
Salad greens, all types

Sweet Substitutes
Gelatin, sugar-free
Jam or jelly, sugar-free
   (2 tsp)
Whipped topping
   (2 Tbsp)
Spreadable fruit,
   no sugar added (1 tsp)

Seasonings can be used as desired. If you are following a low-sodium diet, be sure to read the labels and choose seasonings that do not contain sodium or salt.

Flavoring extracts
   (vanilla, almond,
   butter, etc.)
Garlic or garlic powder
Herbs, fresh or dried
Lemon or lemon juice
Lime or lime juice

Onion powder
Paprika
Pepper
Pimento
Spices
🔖 Soy sauce
Worcestershire sauce

🌿 High in fiber.
🔖 High in sodium.
💧 High in cholesterol.

Meal Plan/1200 Calories
with less than 1200 calories/day may not fulfill nutritional needs.

Carbohydrate:	149 g	49% of total calories
Protein:	61 g	20% of total calories
Fat:	42 g	31% of total calories

These two menus show some of the ways the exchange lists can be used to add variety to your meals.
Use the exchange lists to plan your own menus.

Breakfast

	Sample Menu 1	Sample Menu 2
1 Starch/Bread (List 1)	1/2 cup bran flakes cereal	1/2 bagel (whole wheat or pumpernickel)
1 Fruit (List 4)	1/2 banana	3/4 cup mandarin oranges, drained and mixed with
1 Milk (List 5)	8 oz skim or 1% milk	1 cup lemon nonfat yogurt

Lunch

1 Starch/Bread (List 1)	1 slice whole wheat bread	1 slice rye bread
2 Meat (List 2)	2 oz sliced lean ham	2 oz sliced turkey
0–1 Vegetable (List 3)	Carrot sticks, radishes*	Sliced tomato, lettuce on sandwich*
1 Fruit (List 4)	1 apple	1 1/4 cups watermelon
1 Fat (List 6)	1 Tbsp reduced-calorie mayonnaise OR 1 tsp margarine	1 Tbsp reduced-calorie mayonnaise

Dinner

2 Starch/Bread (List 1)	1 small dinner roll	1 small dinner roll or tortilla
	1/3 cup brown rice	1/2 cup corn or malanga
2 Meat (List 2)	2 oz baked chicken	2 oz flank steak, broiled or grilled
1 Vegetable (List 3)	1/2 cup cooked broccoli	1/2 cup green beans
1 Fruit (List 4)	1 1/4 cups strawberries	1 cup cantaloupe/honeydew melon salad
2 Fat (List 6)	1 tsp margarine	1 tsp margarine for corn
	1 Tbsp regular salad dressing	1 Tbsp slivered almonds for green beans
	Green salad*	

Evening Snack

1 Starch/Bread (List 1)	3 cups hot air popcorn	1 oz (1 1/2 cups) puffed wheat or rice cereal
1 Milk (List 5)	8 oz sugar-free cocoa	8 oz skim or 1% milk

*From List 7—Free Foods

Key: oz. = ounce
       Tbsp = tablespoon
       tsp = teaspoon

Individualized Menu

Calories:	....
Carbohydrate:	....
Protein:	....
Fat:	....

Breakfast   Time:

....

....

....

Lunch   Time:

....

....

....

Dinner   Time:

....

....

....

Evening Snack   Time:

....

Meal Plan/1500 Calories

Carbohydrate: 179 g   48% of total calories
Protein: 74 g   20% of total calories
Fat: 54 g   32% of total calories

These two menus show some of the ways the exchange lists can be used to add variety to your meals.
Use the exchange lists to plan your own menus.

Individualized Menu

Calories: ....
Carbohydrate: ....
Protein: ....
Fat: ....

	Sample Menu 1	Sample Menu 2
Breakfast		
2 Starch/Bread (List 1)	1/2 cup bran flakes cereal	1 bagel (whole wheat or pumpernickel)
	1 slice whole wheat toast	
1 Fruit (List 4)	1/2 banana	3/4 cup mandarin oranges,
1 Milk (List 5)	8 oz skim or 1% milk	drained and mixed with
1 Fat (List 6)	1 tsp margarine	1 cup lemon nonfat yogurt
		1 Tbsp cream cheese

Breakfast   Time:
....
....
....
....
....
....

Lunch		
2 Starch/Bread (List 1)	2 slices whole wheat bread	2 slices rye bread
2 Meat (List 2)	2 oz sliced lean ham	2 oz sliced turkey
0-1 Vegetable (List 3)	Carrot sticks, radishes*	Sliced tomato, lettuce on sandwich*
1 Fruit (List 4)	1 apple	1/4 cups watermelon
1 Fat (List 6)	1 Tbsp reduced-calorie	1 Tbsp reduced-calorie mayonnaise
	mayonnaise	
	OR 1 tsp margarine	

Lunch   Time:
....
....
....
....
....

Dinner		
2 Starch/Bread (List 1)	1 small dinner roll	1 small dinner roll or tortilla
	1/3 cup brown rice	1/2 cup corn or malanga
3 Meat (List 2)	3 oz baked chicken	3 oz flank steak, broiled or grilled
1 Vegetable (List 3)	1/2 cup cooked broccoli	1/2 cup green beans
1 Fruit (List 4)	1 cup raspberries	1 cup cantaloupe/honeydew me on salad
2 Fat (List 6)	1 tsp margarine	1 tsp margarine for corn
	1 Tbsp regular salad dressing	1 Tbsp slivered almonds for green beans
	Green salad*	

Dinner   Time:
....
....
....
....
....

Evening Snack		
1 Starch/Bread (List 1)	3 cups hot air popcorn	1 oz (1 1/2 cups) puffed wheat or rice cereal
1 Milk (List 5)	8 oz sugar-free hot cocoa	8 oz skim or 1% milk

Evening Snack   Time:
....
....

*From List 7—Free Foods

Key: oz = ounce
Tbsp = tablespoon
tsp = teaspoon

Meal Plan/1800 Calories

Carbohydrate:	224 g 50% of total calories
Protein:	90 g 20% of total calories
Fat:	60 g 30% of total calories

These two menus show some of the ways the exchange lists can be used to add variety to your meals.
Use the exchange lists to plan your own menus.

Breakfast

Sample Menu 1

1/2 cup bran flakes cereal
1 slice whole wheat toast
1/2 banana
8 oz skim or 1% milk
1 tsp margarine

2 Starch/Bread (List 1)
1 Fruit (List 4)
1 Milk (List 5)
1 Fat (List 6)

Sample Menu 2

1 bagel (whole wheat or pumpernickel)

3/4 cup mandarin oranges
   drained and mixed with,
1 cup lemon nonfat yogurt
1 Tbsp cream cheese

Lunch

2 Starch/Bread (List 1)
3 Meat (List 2)
0–2 Vegetable (List 3)
1 Fruit (List 4)
1 Fat (List 6)

Sample Menu 1

2 slices whole wheat bread
3 oz sliced lean ham
Carrot sticks, radishes*
1 apple
1 Tbsp reduced-calorie
   mayonnaise
   OR 1 tsp margarine

Sample Menu 2

2 slices rye bread
3 oz sliced turkey
Sliced tomato, lettuce on sandwich*
1/4 cups watermelon
1 Tbsp reduced-calorie mayonnaise

Dinner

3 Starch/Bread (List 1)

3 Meat (List 2)
2 Vegetable (List 3)
1 Fruit (List 4)
2 Fat (List 6)

Sample Menu 1

1 small dinner roll
2/3 cup brown rice
3 oz baked chicken
1 cup cooked broccoli
1 cup raspberries
1 tsp margarine
1 Tbsp regular salad dressing
Green salad*

Sample Menu 2

1 small dinner roll or tortilla
1 cup corn or malanga
3 oz flank steak, broiled or grilled
1 cup green beans
1 cup cantaloupe/honeydew melon salad
2 tsp margarine for corn

Evening Snack

1 Starch/Bread (List 1)
1 Fruit (List 4)
1 Milk (List 5)

Sample Menu 1

3 graham cracker squares
1 small peach or pear
8 oz sugar-free hot cocoa

Sample Menu 2

1 oz (1 1/2 cups) puffed wheat or rice cereal
1/2 banana
8 oz skim or 1% milk

*From List 7—Free Foods

Key: oz = ounce
       Tbsp = tablespoon
       tsp = teaspoon

Individualized Menu

Calories:	....
Carbohydrate:	....
Protein:	....
Fat:	....

Breakfast   **Time:**

....

Lunch   **Time:**

....

Dinner   **Time:**

....

Evening Snack   **Time:**

....

Meal Plan/2000 Calories

Carbohydrate:	246 g	48% of total calories
Protein:	99 g	20% of total calories
Fat:	72 g	32% of total calories

These two menus show some of the ways the exchange lists can be used to add variety to your meals.
Use the exchange lists to plan your own menus.

Breakfast

	Sample Menu 1	Sample Menu 2
2 Starch/Bread (List 1)	1/2 cup bran flakes cereal 1 slice whole wheat toast	1 bagel (whole wheat or pumpernickel)
1 Fruit (List 4)	1/2 banana	3/4 cup mandarin oranges drained and mixed with 1 cup lemon nonfat yogurt
1 Milk (List 5)	8 oz skim or 1% milk	
1 Fat (List 6)	1 tsp margarine	Tbsp cream cheese

Lunch

3 Starch/Bread (List 1)	2 slices whole wheat bread	2 slices rye bread
2 Meat (List 2)	1/2 cup noodles in broth* 2 oz sliced lean ham	1 oz pack tortilla or potato chips 🔲 2 oz sliced turkey
0–1 Vegetable (List 3)	Carrot sticks, radishes*	Sliced tomato, lettuce on sandwich*
1 Fruit (List 4)	1 apple	1 1/4 cups watermelon
1 Milk (List 5)	8 oz skim or 1 % milk	8 oz skim or 1% milk
2 Fat (List 6)	2 Tbsp reduced-calorie mayonnaise OR 2 tsp margarine	Mustard on sandwich* (Fats in chips—see above)

Afternoon Snack

1 Starch/Bread (List 1)	3/4 oz pretzels	8 animal crackers

Dinner

2 Starch/Bread (List 1)	1 small dinner roll	1 small dinner roll or tortilla 1/2 cup corn or malanga
4 Meat (List 2)	1/3 cup brown rice 4 oz baked chicken	4 oz flank steak, broiled or grilled
2 Vegetable (List 3)	1 cup cooked carrots	1/2 cup green beans 1/2 cup mushrooms, sauteed in 1 tsp margarine
1 Fruit (List 4)	1 cup raspberries	1 cup cantaloupe/honeydew melon salad
2 Fat (List 6)	1 tsp margarine 1Tbsp regular salad dressing, Green salad*	1 tsp margarine for corn 1 tsp margarine for mushrooms—see above)

Evening Snack

1 Starch/Bread (List 1)	3 cups hot air popcorn	1 oz (1 1/2 cups) puffed wheat or rice cereal
1 Fruit (List 4)	1 small peach or pear	1/2 banana
1 Milk (List 5)	8 oz sugar-free hot cocoa	8 oz skim or 1% milk

*From List 7—Free Foods   **Key:**   oz = ounce   Tbsp = tablespoon   tsp = teaspoon

---

Individualized Menu

Calories:
Carbohydrate:
Protein:
Fat:

Breakfast .... Time:

....
....
....
....

Lunch .... Time:

....
....
....
....

Afternoon Snack .... Time:

....

Dinner .... Time:

....
....
....
....

Evening Snack .... Time:

....
....
....

Meal Plan/2500 Calories

Carbohydrate: 306 g   49% of total calories
Protein: 122 g   19% of total calories
Fat: 90 g   32% of total calories

These two menus show some of the ways the exchange lists can be used to add variety to your meals.
Use the exchange lists to plan your own menus.

Breakfast

	Sample Menu 1	Sample Menu 2
3 Starch/Bread (List 1)	1/2 cup bran flakes cereal 2 slices whole wheat toast	1 1/2 bagel (whole wheat or pumpernickel)
1 Fruit (List 4)	1/2 banana	3/4 cup mandarin oranges, drained and mixed with
1 Milk (List 5)	8 oz skim or 1% milk	1 cup lemon nonfat yogurt
2 Fat (List 6)	2 tsp margarine	2 Tbsp cream cheese

Lunch

4 Starch/Bread (List 1)	2 slices whole wheat bread, 1/2 cup noodles in broth*, 6 saltine crackers	4 slices rye bread (for 2 sandwiches)
3 Meat (List 2)	3 oz sliced lean ham	3 oz sliced turkey
0–1 Vegetable (List 3)	Carrot sticks, radishes*	Sliced tomato, lettuce on sandwich*
2 Fruit (List 4)	2 Tbsp raisins 1 apple	2 1/2 cups watermelon
1 Milk (List 5)	8 oz. skim or 1% milk	8 oz. skim or 1% milk
2 Fat (List 6)	2 Tbsp reduced-calorie mayonnaise OR 2 tsp margarine	2 Tbsp reduced-calorie mayonnaise

Afternoon Snack

1 Starch/Bread (List 1)	1 pita pocket (4")	8 Melba toast rounds
1 Meat (List 2)	1/4 cup tuna	1 oz. mozzarella string cheese

Dinner

3 Starch/Bread (List 1)	1 small dinner roll 2/3 cup brown rice	small dinner roll or tortilla 1 cup corn or malanga
4 Meat (List 2)	4 oz baked chicken	4 oz flank steak, broiled or grilled
2 Vegetables (List 3)	1 cup cooked broccoli	1/2 cup green beans 1/2 cup mushrooms, sauteed in 1 tsp margarine 1 cup cantaloupe/honeydew melon salad
1 Fruit (List 4)	1 cup raspberries	1 tsp margarine for corn
3 Fat (List 6)	2 tsp margarine 1 Tbsp regular salad dressing Green salad*	1 Tbsp slivered almonds for green beans (1 tsp margarine for mushrooms—see above)

Evening Snack

1 Starch/Bread (List 1)	3 cups hot air popcorn	1 oz (1 1/2 cups) puffed wheat or rice cereal
1 Fruit (List 4)	1 small peach or pear	1/2 banana
1 Milk (List 5)	8 oz sugar-free hot cocoa	8 oz skim or 1% milk

*From List 7—Free Foods   Key: oz = ounce   Tbsp = tablespoon   tsp = teaspoon

Individualized Menu

Calories: ....
Carbohydrate: ....
Protein: ....
Fat: ....

Breakfast .... Time: ....
....
....
....

Lunch .... Time: ....
....
....
....
....

Afternoon Snack .... Time: ....
....

Dinner .... Time: ....
....
....
....
....

Evening Snack .... Time: ....
....
....

5

The Pritikin Program and Diabetes

- Benefits of the Pritikin Program
- The Pritikin Diet
- Special Guidelines for Diabetics

In 1957, Nathan Pritikin was diagnosed with life-threatening heart disease and a high blood-cholesterol level. But in defiance of what was then medical convention, Pritikin decided he would treat himself—with a low-fat, high-fiber diet and regular aerobic exercise. His doctors tried to dissuade him; they believed exercise could kill a man in his condition and that cardiovascular disease bore little or no relation to diet. From the literature on nutrition and heart disease, however, he found data that linked diet and cholesterol. Encouraged, Pritikin set out on a course far more pioneering and promising than any simple diet could provide. He began a new way of eating. He embarked on a daily walking—and, later, jogging—regimen. And he monitored his heart and cholesterol level with batteries of tests. Twelve months later, his blood cholesterol had dropped 140 points. By 1966, his cardiovascular endurance had so improved that he was able to run seven miles a day. His stress tests now showed no evidence of coronary insufficiency. Pritikin had turned his life around. And he felt wonderful.

Nathan Pritikin boosted the country's fitness consciousness when he opened the Pritikin Longevity Center in 1976, thus putting into practice his personal—and clinically tested—philosophy of cardiovascular health resulting from proper nutrition, exercise, and stress management. Many of the ideas that seemed far-fetched when Pritikin first espoused them in the fifties are widely accepted today by the national medical community. Nutritional recommendations from the prestigious American Heart Association, for example, increasingly reflect those outlined in the Pritikin Program. Current research continues to bolster the Pritikin view by establishing connections between cholesterol and cardiovascular disease and by demonstrating the adverse effects of stress and a sedentary lifestyle on well-being.

If you eat the way the average American does, your foods are riddled with fat; high in cholesterol, sodium, and sugar; and low in fiber. High saturated-fat levels contribute to cardiovascular disease, the most common cause of death in the United States. Too much cholesterol can cause coronary artery disease and cerebrovascular disease. (See Chapter 16, *Diabetes, Lipids, and Atherosclerosis*.) An excess of sodium bears a direct relation to elevated blood pressure, another serious health problem. A diet high in refined sugar tends to increase the triglyceride level in the blood. The typical American diet contains too few fresh fruits, vegetables, grains, and legumes, which can help you avoid constipation and other digestive problems and even prevent some forms of cancer.

The Pritikin Program combats these health risks by using a back-to-basics approach. In many ways, this plan reflects the zero-technology foods eaten for thousands of years: unrefined, unprocessed, low-fat, high-fiber foods—

a variety of fresh, wholesome fruits, vegetables, grains, and legumes, and modest amounts of fish, poultry, lean meats, and nonfat dairy products.

The health secret to these foods is that they drastically cut your fat and cholesterol consumption. On your current diet, you're probably getting around 40% of your daily calories in the form of fat. The American Heart Association and other health agencies say that figure is too high. On the Pritikin plan, less than 10% of your daily calories come from fat. In addition, staying away from excess sugar, salt, caffeine, and alcohol can improve your health.

The backbone of the Pritikin food plan is carbohydrates. Seventy-five to eighty percent of your daily calories will be in the form of unrefined carbohydrates (vegetables, fruits, grains, pastas, legumes, breads). These are great energy sources, so you'll have plenty of pep on this plan. And since unrefined carbohydrates (whole-grain bread, brown rice) are emphasized here, your vitamin, mineral, and fiber requirements will be easily satisfied.

The Pritikin Program can improve your health. Stress, exercise, and smoking do influence health, but nutrition is the key to preventing, halting, and even reversing some health problems. Fact: Scientific studies show that the risk of heart attack is reduced when the blood-cholesterol level drops. The Pritikin plan can significantly lower blood-cholesterol levels. Fact: High dietary fiber is believed to help prevent colon and rectal cancer as well as other diseases of the digestive tract. The Pritikin plan is fiber rich. Fact: Weight reduction can significantly reduce blood pressure and the blood-sugar levels of some diabetics. The Pritikin plan can help you lose weight safely.

Being more than just a few pounds overweight increases the risk of degenerative diseases such as adult-onset diabetes, heart disease, hypertension, and breast, uterine, and colon cancer. Research conducted during the Framingham Heart Study found that for each extra pound of weight, the risk of death increased by 2% for non-smokers between the ages of 50 and 62, and by 1% for nonsmokers between the ages of 30 and 49. People about 10% under average weight have the best prospects of all. The overweight have a three times greater risk of hypertension and a one and one-half times greater chance of elevated cholesterol levels.

One goal of the Pritikin plan is to lower and normalize elevated risk factors such as blood-cholesterol and triglyceride (fat) levels, but an additional benefit of the plan often is weight loss. The Pritikin Program offers guidelines for improving your eating habits for the rest of your life. How-to information on weight loss is included. Concentrate on familiarizing yourself with the eating and exercise plan, and be assured that you can shed pounds without having to calculate calories or go hungry . . . ever.

FAT

Food	% of calories from fat
Butter/margarine	100%
Vegetable oil	100%
Mayonnaise	99%
Salad dressing	95%
Coconut	92%
Half-and-half	90%
Cream cheese	90%
Spareribs	80%

CHOLESTEROL

Food	mg of cholesterol
Liver (3.5 oz)	450
Egg yolk (1)	252
Beef, tenderloin (8 oz)	188
Italian sausage (2 links)	130
Cheeseburger (4 oz)	107
Lamb, lean leg (3.5 oz)	99

The charts above depict some of the worst offenders against a healthy eating plan. Choose foods in which fat content is less than 15% of total calories. The exceptions to this 15% rule are foods in the fish, fowl, and meat group, where the maximum is 34%. The foods in the cholesterol chart are among those highest in cholesterol.

Carbohydrates are very important to the Pritikin plan. All carbohydrates are not equally good for you. Choose unrefined carbohydrates, such as whole grains. White bread, white rice, and other refined products have had many of the vitamins and minerals—not to mention the fiber—milled out of them, and pastries are high in fat and loaded with sugar. Don't overlook vegetables, beans, and corn, which are also carbohydrates. These foods plus natural, unrefined grains are at the foundation of the Pritikin Program; they're low in fat, high in vitamins and minerals, and contain moderate amounts of protein. And they're filling without being fattening.

Fiber deserves all the attention it has been getting. No matter what your age, you should be sure you're getting enough of it. Fiber is the indigestible part of plant cells. It adds bulk to waste products passing through your digestive system, speeding elimination of bile acids, which in turn provides protection against colon and rectal cancer, diverticulosis, gallstones, and hemorrhoids. Researchers believe a high-fiber diet keeps blood sugar levels in balance and may therefore help control diabetes. Soluble fiber—the type found in oat bran, legumes (navy, lima, and kidney beans), vegetables (corn), fruits (apples and oranges), and brown rice—actually *lower* cholesterol.

You would probably have to triple the amount of fiber you're currently getting in order to meet the 25 to 35 grams per day standard set by the American Dietetic Association. On the Pritikin Program, you will be assured of at least 40 grams daily. The amount of protein you'll get on the Pritikin Program is the same amount most Americans currently consume—10 to 15% of daily calories. The difference is in the *source* of protein. On the Pritikin Program, most of the protein comes from vegetables, grains, and legumes rather than from animal products. These foods are good sources of protein, and they don't carry the dietary fat and cholesterol of animal products. Protein, which aids tissue repair, is only needed in small amounts. Instead of eating meat as a main course, you'll be eating mostly vegetable and grain entrees, with fish, poultry, and lean meats functioning either as a side dish or condiment in a main dish. To ensure daily cholesterol intake does not exceed 100 milligrams, an amount most people can handle, the Pritikin Program recommends that meat intake be kept to 3.5 ounces daily.

Cutting down on fats won't cause you to miss any essential nutrients. Fat is an important energy source, so you do need some in your diet. But believe it or not, fats occur naturally in small amounts in vegetables, grains, and beans. When these foods are combined with the fish, poultry, or meat in the plan, the body's dietary-fat requirements are easily satisfied.

The largest contribution of dietary fat in most diets comes from butter, margarine, cream, and oils; but meat, eggs, whole milk, nuts, and seeds also are high in fat.

Surprisingly, avocados and olives are two other foods with a high fat content.

Excess dietary fat alarms health watchers because a diet high in saturated fats is a major cause of heart disease and strokes. The Finns, whose diet for many years has been high in saturated fat, have one of the highest rates of heart disease. With our rich diet, we Americans also rank high.

Saturated fats (found in foods derived from animal products, and coconut and palm oils) raise blood-cholesterol levels. Unsaturated fats (vegetable oils, such as corn, peanut, safflower, and olive) may not raise blood-cholesterol levels, but they still contribute to obesity and other health problems. The best policy to take toward fats is a hands-off one. Your body can function in top form with the fats it extracts from natural foods.

Even if you already have evidence of atherosclerosis, it is never too late to lower your cholesterol. By lowering it, you may prevent further development of disease, and in some cases, even reverse the process.

The recommended level for blood cholesterol on the Pritikin Program is 160 milligrams per deciliter of blood, or 100 plus your age, whichever is lower. This figure is based on population studies in nations with a low incidence of cardiovascular disease. Research shows that there is almost no risk associated with a cholesterol level below 150.

This figure is much lower than that generally recommended by physicians. The figure your doctor feels comfortable with is probably based on the American norms, not on an ideal. But the American norms are just too high: half of all American adults have levels above the danger line of 200 milligrams per deciliter set by the National Heart, Lung, and Blood Institute. For your own sake, keep your dietary intake of cholesterol low. On the

Pritikin Program you will be getting 100 milligrams (or less) of cholesterol daily. Compare this with the 400 to 500 milligrams most Americans consume daily.

Diet is one of the most important keys to controlling diabetes. Most diabetics quickly master the art of avoiding sugar and many of the fatty foods they had previously found difficult to resist. The standard diabetic diet is based upon food exchanges, total calories, and proportions of carbohydrates, proteins, and fats as described in Chapter 4. These diets are excellent for most people, particularly young persons. However, there is no emphasis on preventive measures against the long-term degenerative complications of diabetes. The Pritikin approach seeks to combat the "Deadly Quartet"—a constellation of the disorders that are associated with insulin resistance and lead to the long-term complications.

Included in the "quartet" are obesity, hypertension, hypertriglyceridemia, and decreased HDL (dyslipidemia, as discussed in Chapter 16). The "Deadly Quartet" increases the risk of microvascular disease—changes in the small blood vessels (capillaries)—that develops when the blood sugar is chronically uncontrolled. This process will be explored in greater depth in Chapter 16. The Pritikin approach to diabetes emphasizes the importance of preventing and treating obesity associated with Type II diabetes and stresses the importance of diet, exercise, and behavioral changes.

The Pritikin diet emphasizes complex carbohydrates, taking into account the preparation, refining, milling, and breakdown of carbohydrates. The dietary program taught at the Pritikin Longevity Center influences the rapidity of digestion and absorption of nutrients and therefore, the effect of blood sugar levels. Unrefined carbohydrates make the body work harder to refuel itself by requiring physiological processes to gradually convert the complex carbohydrates to simple sugars, a process that maintains a more stable blood glucose pattern.

Researchers refer to a food's immediate, post-meal effect on blood sugar as "glycemic-index." In one study, low glycemic-index wheat flour and potatoes had the same percentage of fat and fiber, but the low glycemic-index foods reduced blood sugar more efficiently by 11–20%.

The ingestion of unrefined carbohydrates makes it easier to lose weight by prolonging the feeling of satiety (fullness) and they are more slowly absorbed, adding to the benefit for stabilizing the blood glucose levels in diabetics.

A high soluble fiber diet content also has the important added benefit of slowing the digestive process, improving insulin sensitivity, and lowering the levels of cholesterol and triglycerides—effects that lower the risk for developing vascular disease.

Pasta and parboiled rice have a glycemic index similar to unrefined foods. They are not high in fiber, but their particular kind of starch does have a similar effect on slowing absorption.

Whole-grain hot cereal is better for diabetics than whole wheat bread. Corn on the cob is better than cornmeal. A fresh apple is better than a dried apple.

Vegetarian chili, split pea, and barley soup as well as corn chowder and lentil soup all contain the right foods; the unrefined carbohydrates and the high soluble fiber meet the criteria for aiding in controlling blood sugar levels. In short, the Pritikin Program may offer protection against the rate of development of many of the long-term complications of diabetes. The Pritikin Program recommends eating five to eight small meals every day rather than two or three large meals. This helps to avoid spikes in blood sugar and seems to control appetite and hunger to a greater degree.

Another mainstay in the Pritikin approach consists of "short bursts" of exercise for those who have been accustomed to a sedentary lifestyle, gradually building up to more vigorous exercise over longer periods of time. The exercise lowers and stabilizes blood sugar, improves glucose tolerance, and reduces insulin resistance. Exercise also facilitates the lowering of cholesterol and triglycerides and raises the "good" cholesterol, HDL, all of significant benefit to the diabetic. The exercise should be regular and sustained. Along with the prescribed diet, it will assist in weight loss in the obese diabetic. Most exercise derives 50% of calories from fat and 50% from carbohydrate. Sustained physical activity will use up fat stores, leading to weight loss.

Moderate activities are preferable because high intensity exercise may release hormones which can raise blood sugar levels. The diabetic's physician, knowing the patient's status regarding possible retinopathy, hypertension, and circulatory problems, can prescribe the best type of exercise for the individual diabetic patient.

The Pritikin Program is *not* for everyone. It requires dedication and dietary sacrifices that many people are unwilling to make. Of course, varying degrees of modification can be incorporated into your diabetes control regimen in consultation with your dietitian and physician. This plan is particularly suitable for obese Type II diabetics who may be able to discontinue their medications after following the program. Everyone presents his own unique requirements. Therefore, before undertaking any radical change in your diet, consult your diabetologist for approval and recommendations.

GUIDELINES: ESPECIALLY FOR DIABETICS
IMPORTANT NUTRITIONAL CONSIDERATIONS

For optimal weight loss, blood glucose control, and to lower triglycerides:

Minimize
Breads   Pita
Crackers   Muffins
Dry cereals   Nonfat potato chips
Bagels

Emphasize
Hot cereals (especially oatmeal), corn, barley, brown rice, beans, peas, lentils, garbanzos
Vegetables (unlimited)

Eat with moderation
Pastas and whole grains
Yams, whole potatoes, and sweet potatoes
Limit whole raw fruit to 3–5 servings a day (best are apples, pears, and berries). Remember that one banana counts as two fruit servings.

Avoid
Fruit juices, fruit concentrates, and dried fruits

Have some vegetable medley and 1–2 cups of vegetable soup as mid-morning snacks.

At lunch and dinner, grab a plate and go to the salad bar first. Eat a good plate of salad before going through the line. Don't skip the steamed vegetables when you go through the line.

Always eat some soup. You may have two plates, one of each kind.

Eat some of the vegetable medley with mustard as part of your afternoon snack.

Don't skip breakfast even if you aren't hungry. Never go hungry.

Food Ideas for Diabetics

Breakfast:

1. Hot cooked cereal (oatmeal, Wheatena, 7-Grain, Kasha). Cook cereal with water and/or nonfat milk. Add fruit such as diced apple, banana, or berries. Sprinkle cinnamon and/or nutmeg. It's delicious!
2. Egg-white omelet (egg whites cooked with your favorite vegetables). Several excellent choices include tomatoes, mushrooms, onions, asparagus, green peas, and/or potatoes. Serve with fresh fruit and nonfat yogurt or cottage cheese.

Lunch/Dinner:

Generous portions of homemade or canned soup (Pritikin, Health Valley Brands). Soups should contain both vegetables and beans.

Large salads with a variety of fresh vegetables such as carrots, tomatoes, bell peppers, and cucumbers. Add chicken breast, grilled or broiled fish, tuna salad prepared with nonfat mayonnaise, and/or beans such as garbanzo, kidney, or lima beans. Use a nonfat salad dressing or balsamic vinegar prepared with mustard and Nutrasweet to taste.

Veggie burgers (Boca Burger™) served with brown rice, whole-grain pasta, baked sweet potato or red new potatoes, salad or steamed vegetables.

Pasta with a marinara sauce. Could add chicken or fish to the meal. Serve with salad and fresh fruit for dessert.

Broiled or grilled fish or chicken (4 ounces), served with steamed new potatoes, vegetables of your choice.

Turkey meatloaf, salmon terrine, or veggie loaf. Serve with salad, soup, or steamed vegetables.

Turkey chili—serve as a meal entree or as an afternoon snack. Can be prepared with or without turkey. Could use extra beans in place of turkey.

Any grain can be used as a meal side dish such as rice, bulgar, quinoa, barley. Any vegetables can be used whether raw, steamed, fresh, or frozen. Soups and salads are recommended to be served with lunch and dinner. Include a protein food with both lunch and dinner such as fish, chicken, veggie burger, beans, peas, or lentils. However, use animal protein only once per day.

Snacks:

Soups, soups, soups!!! Use canned soups if necessary to save time.

Dannon "Light" yogurt—add a banana or other piece of fruit.

Low-sodium V-8 juice

Jell-O (sweetened with Nutrasweet)

Pudding (sweetened with Nutrasweet)

Raw veggies (carrots, cucumbers, bell peppers, bok choy)

Baked sweet potato or yam—serve with applesauce (no sugar) and a dash of cinnamon

"Only a pinch Soups" (add hot water, let sit, stir, and eat). These are available in the health food store or Pritikin Sport Store.

Swiss Miss Hot Cocoa (fat free, sugar free)

Nonfat cottage cheese, add fruit (canned peaches without sugar are great)

Snacks on the Road:

    Low-sodium V-8
    Bananas
    Yogurt

Tuna fish served on 100% rye bread (rye is better on blood sugar). Prepare tuna fish with mayonnaise or nonfat sour cream, spread mustard on the bread.

Miscellaneous

Beverages:

Water (plain, bottled, mineral, or flavored), hot grain beverages (coffee substitutes), vegetable juices, and selected herbal teas (such as peppermint, rose hips, or chamomile).

Optional:

The following may enhance your food plan. If desired, use in moderation.

Egg whites: Up to 7 per week.

Sweeteners: For healthy individuals who choose to use sweeteners, a suggested rule of thumb is 2 tablespoons fruit juice concentrate or 1 tablespoon molasses, honey, or brown sugar, etc., per 1,000 calories per day.

Salt and high-sodium foods, condiments: Avoid added salt, highly salted, pickled, and smoked foods. Limit foods that have more than 1 mg of sodium per calorie so as not to exceed 1,600 mg of sodium per day.

Alcoholic beverages: Use in moderation or not at all. Up to 4 drinks per week. A drink is approximately 4 oz of wine, 12 oz of beer, or 1½ oz of 80-proof liquor.

If you want to lose weight: Go wild on vegetables—eat as much as you want. They're only 25 calories each serving.

If your weight is fine:

Celebrate! Eat as many grains, vegetables, and fruits as you want.

Caution

What if you feel stuck and need to adjust your choices? Enter Category 2: "Caution—The Less the Better." While "Caution" foods are not recommended, this list provides direction when food choices are limited. "Caution" foods are roughly placed in order of decreasing desirability according to the amount and type of fat.

Fruits:

Avocados and olives.

Unsalted Nuts and Seeds:

For example, walnuts, almonds, pumpkin kernels, pecans, pistachios, sunflower seeds, filberts, Brazil nuts, peanuts, cashews, and macadamia nuts.

Low-Fat Dairy (1%):

Low-fat yogurt, low-fat milk, and low-fat cheeses.

Oils High in Monounsaturates:

Canola oil, olive oil, avocado oil, and peanut oil.

Oils High in Polyunsaturates:

Walnut oil, soybean oil, sunflower oil, corn oil, sesame oil, and safflower oil.

Stop

"Stop" means exactly that. When faced with foods in the "Stop" category, search for "Go" and, if necessary, "Caution" foods. These foods, due to their high content of saturated fat, total fat, and/or cholesterol, will significantly compromise the goals of the Pritikin Program.

Animal Fats, Tropical Oils, and Processed Oils:
Butter, coconut oil, palm kernel oil, lard, chicken fat, palm oil, cocoa butter (chocolate), margarine, hydrogenated and partially hydrogenated vegetable oils and shortening.

Meats:
Fatty meats, organ meats, and processed meats.

Whole and Low-Fat Dairy (2% fat or greater):
Cheese, cream, cream cheese, half and half, ice cream, milk, sour cream, and yogurt.

Nuts:
Coconuts.

Miscellaneous:
Egg yolks, deep-fried foods, nondairy whipped toppings, rich desserts, and pastries.

"GO" FOODS: THE PRITIKIN CENTER EATING PLAN

The Daily Five

1. **Choose no more than one fish, poultry, or meat.**
   One serving daily. Choose from fish, lean fowl, or lean

red meat (3^1/$_2$ oz). A serving would be about the size of the palm of your hand and the thickness of a deck of cards. Among the shellfish, keep shrimp to 2 oz.

2. **Choose no more than two dairy foods.** Two servings daily. Choose from nonfat milk (1 cup), nonfat yogurt (^{3}/$_4$ cup), or nonfat cheese (2 oz).

3. **Choose at least three fruits.** Three or more servings of whole fruit daily. For most fruits a serving fits into your hand. Fruit juice (^{1}/$_2$ cup) may be used in place of up to one-third of fruit servings.

4. **Choose at least four vegetables.** Four or *more* servings of raw or cooked vegetables daily. A serving is about 1 cup of raw vegetables or ^{1}/$_2$ cup of cooked vegetables. Include dark green and yellow or orange vegetables daily. You may choose vegetable juice in place of up to one-quarter of your vegetable servings.

5. **Choose at least five whole-grain breads, pastas, and cereals.** Five or *more* servings of whole grains daily (for example, wheat, oats, rye, corn, brown rice, barley, millet) in the form of cereal, side dishes, pasta, or bread. A serving is approximately 80 calories. Also included as options are starchy vegetables like potatoes, yams, and winter squashes or chestnuts, beans, and peas.

Vegetarian Options

Instead of meat, fish, or poultry, substitute either beans, peas, or lentils (^{2}/$_3$ cup), tofu (6 oz), or low-fat cheese (2 oz) with less than 34% of its calories from fat.

6

Insulin

- Sources of Insulin
- Different Types and Mode of Action
- Cautions Regarding Use

People with Type I diabetes can't make their own insulin. They must take insulin injections every day to live.

People with Type II diabetes may make insulin, but they can't use it well. They can survive without insulin injections, but taking insulin often helps them keep their blood sugar closer to normal and to feel better. About 40% of people with Type II diabetes eventually take insulin injections.

Insulin cannot be taken in a pill or tablet form. It must be injected under the skin, using a syringe.

HOW MUCH INSULIN DO YOU NEED?

Each person is different. The amount of insulin you need depends on your:

- body weight
- body build (how much fat and muscle you have)
- level of physical activity
- daily food intake
- other medicines

- emotions
- general health
- amount of stress

HOW MANY TIMES EACH DAY?

Because people can be different in all of the ways listed, their needs for insulin will also be different. People also differ in when they need to take insulin.

- Some people can control their diabetes with only one shot of insulin a day.
- Most people need two or more shots every day to keep their blood sugar in control.
- Some people need more than one *type* of insulin.

THE GOAL IS CONTROL

Taking more shots does not mean your diabetes is worse. Control, not treatment, is the best way to judge how much of a problem your diabetes is. A person with Type II diabetes who takes three shots a day and has near-normal blood sugar is much better off than someone who takes diabetes pills or one shot a day and has high blood sugar.

CHANGING YOUR DOSE(S) AND SCHEDULE

When you first start taking insulin, your doctor will probably change the dose or schedule several times. These changes will be made when your blood sugar tests show that a change is needed. Ask questions. It's important that you understand when and how your particular schedule of insulin works. Follow the doctor's instructions carefully. Together, you and your doctor can find the insulin routine that is best for your needs and lifestyle.

WHERE DOES BOTTLED INSULIN COME FROM?

The label on your insulin bottle shows that the insulin is either human or animal-source insulin. This is called the species of the insulin.

- "Human insulin" does not come from human beings, but is made to be the same as the insulin made by the human body. Human insulin is made in one of two ways:

  1. Recombinant DNA technology, a chemical process that makes it possible to make unlimited amounts of human insulin.
  2. A process that chemically changes pork insulin to make human insulin.

- Beef insulin comes from cows.
- Pork insulin comes from pigs.

TYPES AND ACTIONS OF INSULIN

There is a large letter or number on the label of your insulin bottle. It shows the type of your insulin. The following types of insulin are available in the United States.

R = Regular insulin
S = Semilente insulin

N = NPH insulin
L = Lente insulin
50/50 = 50% NPH and 50% Regular insulin
70/30 = 70% NPH and 30% Regular insulin
U = Ultralente insulin

Knowing an insulin's type will tell you how fast it starts to work and how long it works. This is called its action, or activity.

- Regular and Semilente insulins are short-acting insulins. They start to work quickly and are finished working sooner than other types of insulin.
- NPH and Lente insulins are intermediate-acting insulins. These insulins take longer to start acting than R and S insulins. They also keep working longer than R and S insulins.
- 70/30 insulin combines the actions of R and N insulins. The 30% Regular in the premixed insulin begins to work quickly. The 70% NPH begins to act as the R is finishing. 50/50 insulin has equal parts of Regular and NPH insulins.
- Ultralente insulin is long-acting. It starts very slowly and lasts a longer time.

The following chart shows the duration of activity of some short-acting, intermediate-acting, and long-acting human insulin. All types and species of insulin work in the same way to lower blood sugar.

Duration of Activity of Human Insulins

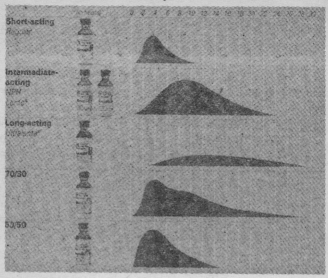

DURATION OF ACTIVITY OF HUMAN INSULIN

Start: The start of the curve (left side) shows how long it usually takes for the insulin to start working.

Peak: The light area in the center of the curve shows when the insulin usually has its strongest effect.

End: The dark area at the end of the curve (right side) shows how long the insulin usually stays in the body.

All of the times shown are estimates. Each insulin may work a little differently in your body. The times of onset, peak, and duration of effect vary greatly among individuals and are affected by many factors, including dose, species, site of injection, exercise of the injection area, and insulin antibodies.

Regular insulin may also be administered intravenously.

HOW MUCH INSULIN IS IN THE BOTTLE

Just as height is measured in inches, insulin is measured in "units." A unit is a small amount of pure insulin. All bottles of insulin sold in the United States have 100 units of insulin in each milliliter of fluid. Such bottles say U-100 on the label. The amount of insulin in a milliliter (U-100) is called the insulin's concentration.

Since each insulin bottle holds 10 milliliters of fluid, a bottle of U-100 insulin contains 1,000 units. Bottles of U-100 insulin have orange caps. (Bottles of U-40 insulin are available in some countries outside the U.S. These bottles have red caps.)

Check the expiration date printed on the insulin box before you buy it. The date must allow enough time for you to use the whole bottle. To find out how long the bottle will need to last, divide the number of units in the bottle by the number of units you take each day.

For example:

1,000 units U-100 divided by 35 units per day = 28 days of insulin. In this case, if you start a new bottle of NPH on March 1, you will finish it on March 28. You should not buy a bottle with an expiration date earlier than March 28.

1,000 units U-100 divided by 15 units per day = 66 days of insulin. In this case, if you start a new bottle of Regular insulin on March 1, you will finish it on May 5. You should not buy a bottle with an expiration date earlier than May 5.

Practice here to find how long a bottle of your insulin will last:

Type of insulin-
Units in bottle   units each day   days of insulin
                                                 for this bottle

1,000 units—   divided by—   =   _____

ADVICE ABOUT BUYING INSULIN AND SYRINGES

When buying insulin, check the insulin box and label carefully. Make sure you get the exact kind of insulin your doctor wants you to take. Using the wrong insulin can affect your diabetes control.

You need to know certain facts about your insulin in order to buy the right kind.

You must know the:

- species (human, beef, pork, or mixed beef-pork)
- brand name (Humulin, Illetin, Illetin II, etc.)
- type (NPH, Regular, Lente, etc.)
- concentration (U-100 is the most common in the U.S.; U-500 is available only by prescription.)

Write the species, brand name, type, and concentration of the insulin(s) you use in the space below:

Species   Brand Name   Type   Concentration

Do not change the species, brand, type, or concentration of your insulin(s) unless you first discuss the change with your doctor. Any change in insulin should be made cautiously and only under medical supervision.

The syringes you buy *must match* the concentration of your insulin. If you use the U-100 insulin, your syringe should have orange tops and say U-100 on the package.

CHECK YOUR INSULIN BEFORE YOU USE IT

Before using your insulin, look at it carefully. If insulin doesn't look right, it may not work right. Regular insulin should be clear and have *no color*. Do not use Regular insulin if it looks cloudy, thickened, even slightly colored, or if it has any solid particles in it.

All other insulins should have an even, cloudy appearance after gentle shaking—they look a lot like skim milk.

Do not use Semilente, NPH, Lente, 70/30, 50/50, or Ultralente insulins if:

- insulin stays at the bottom of the bottle after gentle shaking.
- there are clumps of insulin in the liquid or on the bottom after gentle shaking.
- solid particles of insulin stick to the bottom or sides of the bottle after gentle shaking. This makes the bottle look "frosted" on the inside.

If your insulin doesn't look right, don't use it. Take it back to your pharmacy.

7

Preparing and Injecting Insulin

- **Insulin Syringes**
- **Injection Sites**
- **Antiseptic Techniques**
- **Preparation of Mixture**

These instructions explain how to draw insulin into a syringe and give yourself an injection.

 1. Wash your hands.

 2. Gently mix the insulin. You can mix it by rolling the bottle between the palms of your hands, by turning the bottle over from end to end a few times, or by shaking the bottle gently.

 3. If this is a new bottle of insulin, remove the flat, colored cap. Do not remove the rubber stopper or the metal band under the cap. Clean the rubber stopper with an alcohol swab.

 4. Remove the cover from the needle. Pull the plunger back until the tip of the plunger is at the line for _____ (X) units. This will pull air into the syringe.

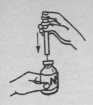

5. Push the needle through the rubber stopper. Press in the plunger to push the air into the bottle of insulin.

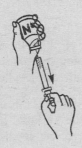

6. Turn the bottle and syringe upside down. Hold the bottle with one hand. The tip of the needle should be in the insulin. Use the other hand to pull back on the plunger until its tip is at the line for _____ (X) units. This will pull insulin into the syringe.

7. Look at the insulin in the syringe. Are there any air bubbles? If so, use the plunger to push the insulin back into the bottle. Then slowly pull insulin into the syringe again. Pull the plunger back to the line for your dose of insulin. Repeat this until there are no large air bubbles in the syringe.

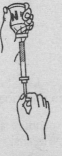

8. Make *sure* the tip of the plunger is at the line for the number of units to be injected. Double-check your dose. Magnifiers that connect to your syringe are available if needed. They can help you see the lines on the syringe more clearly.

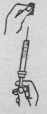

9. Pull the needle out of the rubber stopper. (If you need to lay the syringe down before taking the injection, put the cover back on the needle to protect it.)

10. Now you are ready to give yourself an injection.

INJECTING YOUR INSULIN

These instructions explain how to inject your insulin dose (single or mixed dose). Choose a site for your injection. Each shot should be given in a different spot.

1. Clean the skin at the place for injection with an alcohol swab.

2. Pinch up a large area of skin. Push the needle into the skin, going straight in at a 90 degree angle. Be sure the needle is "way in."

3. Pull back slightly on the syringe. If blood comes into the syringe, the needle has entered a blood vessel. Remove the needle and put it in another location.

4. Push the plunger all the way down. This will push the insulin into your body. Release pinched skin.

5. Pull the needle straight out. Don't rub the place where you gave the injection.

6. Safely dispose of used needles and syringes. Your doctor, pharmacist, or diabetes educator can show you how.

PREPARING A MIXED DOSE OF INSULIN

Many people with diabetes take more than one type of insulin. Two kinds of insulin can be put into the same syringe. This is called a mixed dose of insulin. Mixing should be done just before you take your shot. The following example will show you how to mix two types of insulin in one injection.

Before you try to mix insulin, you should know how to handle syringes and insulin.

If you have not been taking insulin, practice by preparing several single doses of insulin (as described previously) before trying to prepare a mixed dose.

Write your dose of short-acting insulin in units:

_____ (A)

Write your dose of intermediate or longer-acting dose:

_____ (B)

Then, add the total dose together:

_____ (A+B) units

1. Clean the tops of both bottles with an alcohol swab.

2. Inject the _____ (B) units of air into the longer-acting insulin bottle. Do not pull insulin into the syringe. Take the needle out of the bottle.

3. Inject the _____ (A) units of air into the short-acting insulin bottle. Turn the bottle and syringe upside down. Hold the bottle with one hand and use the other hand to pull back on the plunger until you have the number of _____ (A) units of short-acting insulin in the syringe. Be sure to remove any large air bubbles.

4. Gently roll or shake the longer-acting insulin bottle until it is mixed.

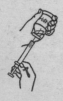

5. Insert the needle into the bottle of longer-acting insulin. Turn the bottle and syringe upside down. Hold the bottle with one hand and use the other hand to pull back slowly on the plunger. Pull the plunger back until you have a total amount of insulin equal to (A)+(B) units in the syringe. Be careful not to push any of the shorter-acting insulin into the longer-acting insulin bottle. (If you pull too much of the longer-acting insulin into the syringe, do not put insulin back into the bottle. Instead, discard the dose and begin again with an empty syringe.)

6. Remove the needle from the bottle. Give the injection of insulin as described in the preceding section.

CHOOSING THE SITE FOR AN INSULIN INJECTION

Choosing exactly where on your body you will give the injection each day is very important.

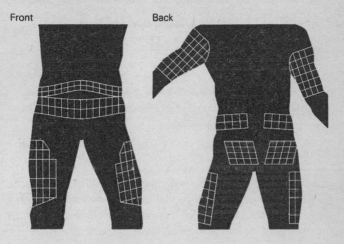

Front   Back

Insulin injection areas

The boxed areas or drawings show suitable sites for your insulin shots. You may need a family member to give you the injection in some of the areas. Each square is an injection site, an exact place to give the shot. To keep skin, fat, and muscle healthy, use a different site for each injection.

Note: Do not inject insulin into an area where the muscles will be exercised vigorously shortly thereafter. For example: avoid the legs prior to jogging.

8

Self-Monitoring of Blood Glucose (SMBG) and Laboratory Testing for Glycosylated Hemoglobin

- Finger-Stick Method
- Glycosylated Hemoglobin
- Equipment

Since the early 1980s, self-monitoring of blood glucose (SMBG) has been shown to be the best way to determine if the blood sugar levels of a person with diabetes mellitus are too high or too low. The development of SMBG is, perhaps, the most significant advance in the treatment of diabetes since the discovery of insulin. Every diabetic should take advantage of it. The measurement helps you to monitor your diabetes control to determine if adjustments in diet, insulin, or exercise are needed. Although SMBG may at first seem difficult and adds to the expense of treatment, diabetes management has improved greatly since this testing method became widely available.

SMBG enables you to become a full partner with your diabetic educator in the management and treatment of your diabetes. Home-monitoring records help your doctor to evaluate your disease and reduce the risks of acute and long-term complications. SMBG enables you to participate fully in everyday activities and control your life without underlying fear and apprehension. By keeping the blood sugars within an optimal range (adjusting insulin dosage, diet, and physical activity), you will have a greater sense of well-being, more stamina, and more energy. By keeping tabs on blood sugar, you will be able to avoid the more obvious symptoms of uncontrolled diabetes, such as excessive thirst, frequency of urination, sweating, fatigue, blurring of vision, and nausea.

The first step in SMBG is to obtain a drop of blood. Fortunately, finger-sticking has become relatively easy and painless with the use of automatic finger-sticking devices. These devices are powered by a spring or jet which thrusts the sharp point of a lancet into the surface of your skin to a predetermined depth in order to draw a drop of blood.

When you are ready to start monitoring, make sure you have all the necessary supplies within reach: a bottle of reagent strips, finger-sticking device with lancet, facial tissues, test strips, and a glucose meter, if you use an electronic device. Before you stick your fingertip, wash your hand with soap and water and then rinse and dry it. Shake your hand a number of times to increase blood flow. Place the finger-sticking device on the tip of your finger. Aim for the side of the finger since this area has fewer pain-feeling nerve endings. Press the release button to puncture the skin. Do not milk or squeeze your finger, since this will mix tissue fluid with the blood. You may apply pressure to the palm of the hand if a large enough drop does not appear.

Many people who do SMBG are instructed to wipe off the first drop of blood (which may be diluted with tissue fluids) and use the second drop. Apply this large drop (don't be stingy) to the reagent pad. While some patients still use the original visual test strip method, most prefer the newer and more reliable hand-held portable electronic meters. The latter are pocket-sized devices that measure the blood glucose and provide a digital readout on a small screen. If you are using a meter, follow the manufacturer's directions carefully.

Generally all that is involved is waiting the appropriate number of seconds and blotting your test strip dry with a facial tissue. Each type of test strip will specify how long to wait before blotting. Next, insert the test strip into the glucose meter. Some will prompt you with beeps to indicate when to do this. Next, wait until the blood glucose measurement appears on the display screen. If you are doing a visual reading, check the reacted portion of the strip against the color chart and determine the closest color match-up. If the color on the strip does not completely match, you must estimate between the higher and lower color chart sample to get an approximation of your blood glucose level.

Some meters can store the results of a large number of tests in a computer memory and provide the doctor with a printed readout of the results. Mistakes include incomplete coverage of the testing pad with blood and negligence in cleaning the meter. Special glucose "control solutions" are available in the newer meters that allow you to test the accuracy of the meter from time to time. The blood strips should be kept in a cool, dry location. Tests with the new meters have shown them to be accurate within 10–15% of commercial laboratory determinations.

GLYCOSYLATED HEMOGLOBIN—ALSO KNOWN AS HEMOGLOBIN A1C

Hemoglobin is the blood substance within the red blood cells that carries oxygen from the lungs to all parts of the body and then removes carbon dioxide formed by the body's metabolism. Red blood cells have a life span of approximately four months. As the red blood cells mature and die, the body constantly forms new ones. Most of the hemoglobin in the red blood cells exists in a form called Hemoglobin A. Normally, a small amount of Hemoglobin A is converted to a different form called Hemoglobin A1c or glycosylated hemoglobin. This occurs when blood glucose attaches to the hemoglobin inside the red blood cell. The chemical union is sometimes written in an abbreviated symbolic form, HbA1c. The amount of glucose that becomes glycosylated depends directly upon the amount of glucose in the blood. High levels of blood glucose sustained over a period of time allow more glucose to become bonded to hemoglobin molecules. Thus, the percentage of hemoglobin that is glycosylated in red blood cells is directly related to the *time* it has been exposed to a given concentration of glucose.

The immediate practical significance of this test is the ability to assess long-term glucose control. The HbA1c level provides information that helps to estimate your average blood glucose level over the previous eight to twelve weeks prior to the test.

HbA1c provides a better index of blood sugar over two to three months than daily (incidental) blood sugar determinations. HbA1c is expressed as a percentage of the total hemoglobin that has glucose attached. The normal range for the HbA1c test is 6% or less. An average blood sugar over a several month period of 120 mg/dl would correspond approximately to a HgA1c of 6%. A reading of 150 mg/dl over the same period would show a reading of about 7%, and 180 mg/dl would be associated with a reading in the 8% range. Readings between 6% and 7% are generally deemed to be acceptable. Readings of 8% or higher are considered undesirable and unacceptable.

It is not a desirable practice to check blood sugar and

give a dose of regular insulin to "cover" a high reading. Checking the urine for ketones should alleviate any concern that the high blood sugar heralds impending acidosis.

For good control, it must be understood that the initial blood sugar in the morning represents the long-acting insulin taken the night before, except when altered by the Somogyi Effect. A swing to a high glucose level in the blood, from an extremely low level, is called the Somogyi Effect. This phenomenon usually occurs at night during sleep. It is due to the release of stress hormones that are secreted to counter the low glucose level. This counter-regulatory mechanism may cause the blood sugar to soar. Those who experience a Somogyi reaction may be completely unaware of their nocturnal hypoglycemic episode. In the morning, when the blood is tested, a high level is noted, leading them to believe they may need more insulin with their evening dose. In fact, the reverse is true. People who experience high glucose levels in the morning need to test their blood sugar in the middle of the night to rule out a Somogyi Effect. This is easily done by keeping the test meter at the bedside and setting an alarm clock for 3 A.M. If blood glucose levels are falling or low, adjustments in the evening snack or insulin dose may be in order. This condition is named for Dr. Michael Somogyi, who first described this phenomenon that is also referred to as the "rebound" effect.

Late afternoon blood sugar represents the action of intermediate insulin taken before breakfast. If the high blood sugar is persistent at a given hour, the patient must consult his doctor to make changes in the intermediate or long-acting insulin (or mixtures of insulin) rather than "treating" the high blood sugar with a dose of fast-acting regular insulin. *So-called "spikes" of sugar do not require treatment immediately with regular insulin.* If each spike is treated with insulin in this manner, the patient may find himself on a self-imposed roller-coaster ride with the sugar going up and down and out of control.

For patients using only one dose of insulin daily to control their blood sugar, before-meal and bedtime testing will usually provide their doctor with adequate information to properly adjust insulin dosage.

Many physicians recommend different regimens for checking blood sugar, depending on food intake, snacks, physical activity, school or work hours, etc.

The main goal is to keep your blood sugar within the range prescribed by your diabetic educator or physician.

For those patients who do not require insulin injections, the morning test can be helpful in estimating rises in blood sugar during the nighttime hours. Another finger-stick an hour after dinner gives information regarding the blood sugar levels during the day.

Without monitoring the blood sugar, one cannot really evaluate diabetic control, the key to reducing long-term complications. Unless the blood sugar can be kept within an acceptable range, there is likely to be slow but steady damage to vital body organs.

Some patients are under the mistaken impression that a blood sugar done in a doctor's office once every three or four weeks is adequate to assess control and prevent the long-term complications described in Chapter 17. This concept is completely erroneous. Frequent monitoring of blood sugars and following hemoglobin HbA1c levels are the only acceptable methods of obtaining reliable data to evaluate diabetes control.

If the finger-stick blood sugar is over 240 mg/dl, the urine should be tested for ketones.

Testing the urine for glucose has been shown to be unreliable for obtaining accurate information regarding blood sugar because the renal threshold (the point above which the urine will contain sugar) varies from individual to individual. In children, the renal threshold is usually low. In older individuals, the renal threshold may run as high as 180 to 190 mg/dl. When the blood glucose rises to abnormally high levels, the kidneys lose the ability to recycle the sugar back into the bloodstream and the sugar literally "spills" into the urine and is excreted. While the renal threshold varies from patient to patient, in general, the sugar is already too high when the urine tests are positive for glucose. For this reason, *blood sugar analysis* has been accepted as the only accurate way to evaluate the management of diabetes.

If your physician is not available and adjustment of your insulin is indicated, two basic facts regarding insulin action must be considered. Regular insulin acts for about 4–6 hours after being administered, reaching its peak action in 2–4 hours. Intermediate-acting insulin (NPH or Lente) continues to have its effect on blood sugar for 10–12 hours and has a peak activity about 6–8 hours after injection. By understanding these two fundamental facts about the action of insulin, excellent control can usually be obtained until you receive further instructions from your doctor or diabetic educator. However, try not to break rule No. 1: *Do not change the amount of your medications on your own. Always consult with your doctor if you think a change is in order.*

EQUIPMENT

Many different brands of meters are currently available. They are all capable of giving accurate information and good service. Some are more convenient than others and some are more complex and expensive. Ask your doctor or diabetic educator what they recommend. If they have no personal preferences you must decide for yourself which one of the products suits your needs best. Shop around before you purchase a meter. Look for a diabetes-supply house or pharmacy that will provide personal instruction in operating the instrument. Also consider test strip costs and availability.

Records of your blood sugar results should be kept and shown to your doctor during your regular visits.

Keeping blood sugar in prescribed ranges as recommended by your physician is the main treatment goal. SMBG helps you to decide if future changes in your activity or insulin routine are indicated.

SMBG has brought an important advance in the management of diabetes that has allowed the patient to "take charge" of his diabetes.

9

Hypoglycemia

- Causes of Low Sugar Reactions
- How to Recognize Hypoglycemia
- Importance of Early Treatment
- Comparison of Diabetic Coma and Insulin Reactions

The word *hypoglycemia* literally means too little sugar in the blood to meet the metabolic needs of the body. Just as the exact level of sugar in the blood varies constantly throughout the day, the body's need for sugar also varies. For this reason, we cannot assign an exact number in milligrams of glucose/dl that will induce symptoms of hypoglycemia in an individual patient. Furthermore, no two people are exactly alike; some will experience the effects of hypoglycemia at levels above "normal" while others will not be symptomatic even at very low levels. Additionally, symptoms of hypoglycemia may be felt when blood sugar levels drop too fast even though blood sugars may remain within the normal range. For this reason, the doctor and the patient must focus on the *clinical* features to determine whether the symptoms being experienced are those of mild, moderate, or severe hypoglycemia. Mild episodes typically produce adrenergic and cholinergic symptoms such as palpitations (awareness of the heartbeat), tachycardia (rapid heart action), pallor, sweating, paresthesias (abnormal sensations of the skin), shakiness, and hunger. Moderate hypoglycemia is likely to hinder concentration. Hypoglycemia may cause an individual to become confused and unable to make rational decisions. Impairment of the function of the brain and central nervous system occurs because the brain relies solely on glucose for its normal metabolic functions. Severe hypoglycemia is characterized by incapacitation, disorientation, seizures, and loss of consciousness. A patient may suddenly develop moderate or severe hypoglycemia within a very short time. Almost all diabetic patients run a risk of hypoglycemia, but it is far more prevalent in those who require insulin for their diabetic management. The majority of episodes occur at night because the body's need for insulin decreases during the predawn hours. It is at this time that the intermediate-acting insulins reach their peak action, causing the blood glucose to drop to low levels. Patients who have elected to follow an intensive insulin regimen or those on the insulin pump run a higher risk for hypoglycemic episodes than patients on conventional therapy.

Insulin is not the only hormone manufactured by the pancreas. Glucagon is another hormone that is secreted when needed, after being manufactured by specific cells called "alpha cells." Glucagon releases sugar (stored as glycogen) from the liver by "breaking down" the glycogen into glucose. Glucagon can raise the blood glucose level temporarily to the point where the unconscious hypoglycemic patient will usually awaken and be able to take nourishment.

When the blood sugar drops below a certain level, depending on the individual patient, the body attempts to compensate by releasing counter-regulatory hormones, primarily glucagon and epinephrine, both of which stimulate glycogen breakdown and release of sugar from the liver.

Some patients have a diminution in the function of this counter-regulatory system and thus may develop severe hypoglycemia without first experiencing symptoms. It is extremely important for these patients to monitor their blood sugar more often and may require raising the usual fasting blood sugar goal of 80–120 mg/dl to approximately 100–140 mg/dl.

The low limits of normal blood sugar range from 55 mg % to 60 mg %. The normal fasting blood sugar ranges from 65 to 115 mg %. In some instances, the failure of the patient to "feel" symptoms of hypoglycemia may result from nerve tissue damage, one of the complications of diabetes. (See Chapter 17, *Long-Term Complications of Diabetes*.)

Patients who have been diagnosed as having diabetes should also be aware that causes and conditions other than diabetes may be responsible for low blood sugar levels. Notable among these are alcohol-induced hypoglycemia, some over-the-counter as well as prescription medications, liver disease, and, rarely, tumors of the pancreas. We shall limit our discussion in this chapter, however, to the most common causes associated with diabetes, namely, low blood sugar resulting from overtreatment with insulin or oral hypoglycemic agents, insufficient food intake, or unscheduled exercise.

Low blood sugar may cause any or all of the following symptoms, depending upon the individual response and the severity of the condition.

1. Hunger
2. Nervousness and irritability
3. Headache
4. Dizziness
5. Faintness
6. Trembling
7. Cold sweat
8. Numbness and tingling around the lips

 9. Difficulty in speaking clearly or slurring of speech
10. Staggering gait
11. Blurred vision
12. Mental confusion
13. Loss of consciousness

Some of these symptoms can be mistaken for other conditions. For example, a diabetic in urgent need of medical care may be mistaken for an intoxicated individual. Alcohol, by itself, can lower blood sugar levels in non-diabetics as well as in diabetics, although its effect on the latter may be particularly severe. Thus a diabetic who is slightly "tipsy" may experience hypoglycemia, requiring treatment, but be neglected because his symptoms are dismissed as purely those of inebriation. This danger makes it advisable to wear a diabetic medic-alert bracelet or pendant. In addition, a wallet-size diabetic identification and information card should be kept on your person.

Low blood sugar can result from one or more of the following situations:

1. Too much medication.
2. The administrations of regular instead of long-acting insulin or the injection of too much insulin by mistake.
3. The skipping or delaying of a regular meal.
4. The skipping of a prescribed between-meal snack.
5. Nausea and vomiting without replacement of food and fluids.
6. The excessive utilization of sugar from unscheduled or excessive physical activity.
7. Drug interactions (certain medications may potentiate the blood lowering of insulin or anti-diabetic oral agents. See page 95).

Patients should familiarize themselves with the properties of the type of insulin prescribed by their doctor and know its mode of action as well as the timing of its peak activity.

TYPES OF INSULIN ACTION

1. Short-Acting:
   Therapeutic action onset: 15–30 minutes
   Peak: 2–4 hours, duration 6–8 hours

2. Intermediate-acting:
   Therapeutic action onset: 2 hours
   Peak: 4–12 hours, duration 10–14 hours

3. Long-Acting:
   Therapeutic action onset: 8 hours
   Peak: 18 hours, duration 24–36 hours

Reactions tend to occur just before a meal or when insulin has a peak effect. The intermediate-acting insulin most often causes reactions in the late afternoon or just before the evening meal. Intermediate-acting insulin taken in the evening can cause reactions during the night or early the next morning.

The education of the diabetic patient includes learning that hypoglycemia may result from sudden changes in insulin dosage, straying from dietary planning, or performing excessive physical activity or exercise. The patient should not hesitate to start treatment after becoming aware of early symptoms of low blood glucose. The hypoglycemia may become severe enough to prevent rapid determination of blood glucose.

IMPORTANT: Diabetics must always carry some form

of carbohydrate, such as hard candy, with them at all times. At the first sign of a possible low blood sugar reaction, even if in doubt, the carbohydrate should be taken.

Quick sources of carbohydrate to treat hypoglycemia include $1/2$ cup of fruit juice, 2 tablespoons of raisins, 5 Life Savers, 6 ounces of milk, $3/4$ cup of non-diet cola, or 5-gram Glucose Tabs. Following the rapid response to glucose, a complex carbohydrate snack is recommended. Milk is the preferred treatment of hypoglycemia in pregnant diabetic patients because of the danger to the fetus from markedly elevated blood sugars.

In the event of a serious hypoglycemic reaction, it is important to keep an injectable vial of *glucagon* on hand that can be administered subcutaneously by members of the family familiar with its use. Complete instructions for its use are in the container that comes with the glucagon vial. The expiration date on the glucagon vial should be checked regularly. It is a good idea to have family members practice using normal sterile saline at intervals so that they are ready and capable should the need arise. If a rapid response to the above measures is not forthcoming, the patient must be taken immediately to the nearest hospital facility for intravenous glucose therapy by trained emergency personnel. Patients on oral medications should be aware that hypoglycemia may last for several hours, and even days in the case of chlorpropamide. This requires constant blood glucose monitoring and intravenous infusion of a glucose solution, especially in older patients.

Patients who reside alone sometimes take too much carbohydrate to offset the symptoms of low blood sugar. Overtreatment can become a problem, causing the patient's sugar to rise to unacceptably high levels.

If the hypoglycemic symptoms are mild, some form of carbohydrate or protein may be able to maintain blood sugar until the next scheduled meal. For example, a glass of milk or slice of cheese should prove adequate, since protein is slowly converted to sugar by the body in sufficient quantities to supply the body with glucose until the next meal.

Hypoglycemia is a complication of diabetes, but with intelligent preparation, knowledge, and adherence to basic principles, it can be managed very well by the vast majority of diabetic patients.

COMPARISON OF DIABETIC COMA & INSULIN REACTIONS

	DIABETIC COMA	INSULIN SHOCK—HYPOGLYCEMIA— LOW BLOOD SUGAR	
	Clinical Features	Regular Insulin	Long-Acting Insulin
Onset	Slow, days	Sudden, minutes	Gradual, hours
Causes	Ignorance and neglect Intercurrent disease Omission of insulin and food	Overdosage Delayed, omitted, or lost meals Excessive exercise before meals	Overdosage Delayed, omitted, or lost meals Excessive exercise before meals
Symptoms	Thirst Frequent urination Headache Nausea Vomiting Abdominal pain Dim vision Constipation Shortness of breath	"Inward nervousness" Weakness Sweating Hunger Double vision, blurred vision Tingling sensations Patient may act drunk Stupor, convulsions	Fatigue Weakness Headache Sweating sometimes absent Dizziness Double, blurred vision Patient may act intoxicated Stupor, convulsions

	Clinical Features	Regular Insulin	Long-Acting Insulin
Signs	Florid face Rapid breathing Dehydration—dry skin Fever Rapid pulse Soft eyeballs Acetone breath Drowsiness Coma	Pallor Shallow respiration Sweating Pulse normal Eyeballs normal	Pallor Shallow respiration Skin may be dry Pulse not characteristic Eyeballs normal
Urine Sugar	Positive	Usually absent, especially in second voided specimen	Usually absent, especially in second voided specimen
Acetone	Positive	Negative	Negative
Diacetic Acid	Positive	Negative	Negative
What to do	Call physician or emergency hospital at first sign of symptoms	If patient is able to swallow, give sugar in some form—candy, syrup, cola or similar beverages that contain sugar, orange juice, etc. Call a physician or emergency hospital.	If patient is able to swallow, give sugar in some form—candy, syrup, cola or similar beverages that contain sugar, orange juice, etc. Call a physician or emergency hospital.
Response to treatment	Slow	Usually rapid	May be slow or late

Note: Excessive dosage of some of the oral hypoglycemic agents or omission of food may cause hypoglycemia, and the symptoms may be the same as those seen with Regular Insulin or the longer-acting insulins.

10

Oral Drugs for Diabetes

- Indications for Use
- Sulfonylureas
- Biguanides

Medications taken by mouth to treat diabetes are known as oral hypoglycemic agents. This is a misnomer, because these medications are not given to cause hypoglycemia— low blood sugar. They are prescribed to *lower* the level of blood glucose to normal or near-normal levels.

The oral drugs that lower the blood sugar *are not insulin.* Although the sugar-lowering effect of some medications as well as certain herbs and plants had been recognized for many years, it was not until World War II that sulfa drugs were noted to have the side effect of lowering blood sugar levels. By the mid-fifties, sulfonylureas were developed specifically for their effect on lowering blood sugar in Type II diabetes. These drugs soon became the treatment of choice for maturity-onset patients who were unable to bring their diabetes under control with diet, weight loss, and exercise programs. The sulfonylurea drugs are most effective in treating Type II diabetes because they work primarily by stimulating the release of insulin from the beta cells of the pancreas. They are far less effective in Type I diabetes because of the inability of the pancreas to produce insulin in these patients. The sulfonylureas are most effective in patients with Type II diabetes with fasting blood sugars below 225 mg/dl. However, there is no universal agreement among diabetologists on this cutoff value.

There are many oral hypoglycemics currently available and all have their own individual characteristics. Some are short-acting, some are intermediate, and others are long-acting. The exact oral medication and dosage to be employed depends on many factors:

1. Body build (height and weight)
2. Type of food intake and adherence to appropriate diet
3. Between-meal snacks
4. Physical activity
5. Response to diet control
6. Response to a particular pill
7. Amount of medication required to achieve normalization of blood sugar
8. Compliance with diet and taking of prescribed medication regularly

During periods of stress, such as an accident or infection, it may be necessary to temporarily stop the oral medicine and control the blood sugar with insulin injections. When the stress is no longer present, the patient usually can go back to the oral agents.

Chlorpropamide (Diabenese) may sometimes cause a severe reaction, with headache and flushing, when taken along with alcoholic beverages. This is called the *antabuse* effect. This phenomenon is also seen on rare occasions with other sulfonylurea drugs.

Low blood sugar reactions can occur with the sulfonylurea oral drugs but usually not with the same severity and frequency as reactions associated with insulin use. However, the same precautions should be adhered to as outlined in Chapter 9, *Hypoglycemia.*

Hypoglycemia occurs most frequently with the intermediate or long-acting preparations. It may be precipitated by skipping meals, liver or kidney disease, concurrent medications that may potentiate the glucose-lowering effect of the sulfonylureas, or from debility. To prevent hypoglycemia, these medications should be started at low dose levels and gradually increased until satisfactory blood sugar control is achieved. Other side effects seen with these drugs are skin rashes and gastro-intestinal symptoms including nausea, vomiting, diarrhea or constipation, heartburn, and flatulence. Abnormalities in liver function and jaundice are occasionally noted. Blood changes rarely seen include low white blood cell counts, anemia, low platelet counts, and, rarely, inhibition of white blood cell production (agranulocytosis).

In some patients, even maximum doses of sulfonylureas prove to be ineffective, a condition that is called primary therapeutic failure. Other patients experience secondary failure: the medication is initially effective, but fails to produce a satisfactory blood sugar lowering effect after several months or years. The percentage of "secondary" failures on sulfonylureas varies from 25 to 30%. In the event of failure, the physician will re-evaluate the patient's adherence to diet and other adjunct measures and may elect to add insulin or a new oral drug for diabetes, metformin. Studies have shown that metformin works synergistically with the sulfonylureas in many cases. This means that although either drug alone might not be adequate to control blood sugar, together their effect is amplified, and they accomplish the therapeutic goal.

Many medications may potentiate the sugar-lowering effect of the sulfonylureas. It is important therefore to inform your diabetologist of any other prescribed drugs or over-the-counter medications that you may be taking.

Beta-blockers mask the signs and symptoms of hypoglycemia and should not be prescribed for patients with diabetes.

Drugs That May Cause Hypoglycemia

Alcohol
Allopurinol (Zyloprim)
Beta-blockers
Clofibrate (Abifrate, Atromid-S)
Coumadin
Fenfluramine (Pondimin)
Monoamine oxidase inhibitors
Probenecid (Benemid)
Salicylates
Sulfonamides (rarely, e.g. Bactrim)

Drugs That May Cause Hyperglycemia

Calcium channel blockers
Corticosteroids
Diazoxide (Proglycem)
Isoniazid
Levothyroxine, etc. (other thyroid hormones)
Nasal decongestants containing epinephrine-like drugs
Oral contraceptives
Dilantin
Rifampin
Thiazide diuretics

Note: Drug interactions vary from person to person. Check your blood sugar more frequently whenever adding or discontinuing any medication.

ORAL HYPOGLYCEMIC AGENTS

First-Generation Sulfonylurea Drugs

Generic name	*Trade Name*	*Duration of Action*
Tolbutamide Dose: 500–1500 mg/day	Orinase	6–12 hours. Metabolized by the liver and excreted in the urine, as are all the sulfonylureas.
Tolazamide Dose: 100–500 mg/day	Tolinase	12–24 hours. Less likely to cause water retention because of its diuretic properties.
Clorpropamide Dose: 100–250 mg/day	Diabenese	Effect may last as long as three days. Can increase secretion of anti-diuretic hormone resulting in water retention and abnormal lowering of sodium in the blood.
Acetohexamide Dose: 250–500 mg/day	Dymelor	12–24 hours

Second-Generation Sulfonylurea Drugs

These drugs are more potent than the first-generation sulfonylureas and therefore require lower doses and have fewer side effects. Adverse reactions are seen in less than 2% of those taking these medications, an incidence less than half that of their predecessors. These are:

Generic name	*Trade Name*	*Duration of Action*
Glipizide Dose: 5–20 mg/day	Glucatrol Glucatrol XL	12–24 hours

Generic name	Trade Name	Duration of Action
Glyburide	Diabeta, Micronase, Glynase	12–24 hours

Dose: 1.5–20 mg/day
Glynase Dose: 3–10 mg/day

Third-Generation Sulfonylurea Drugs

Generic name	Trade Name	Duration of Action
Glimepiride	Amaryl	24 hours

Dose: Starting dose 1 mg/day; usual maintenance dose 1–4 mg/day. Maximum dose: 8 mg/day

Amaryl is insulin sparing and controls glucose without any significant increase in fasting insulin levels. It is indicated for use alone as well as second-line in combination with insulin. Amaryl binds to a different part of the sulfonylurea cell receptors than other drugs in this group. The clinical relevance of this mechanism has not yet been established. The combined use of Amaryl and insulin may increase the potential for hypoglycemia.

Biguanides

Generic name	Trade Name	Duration of Action
Metformin	Glucophage	4–8 hours

Dose: 500–2,000 mg (rarely 2,500 mg)

Metformin is a new drug that is having a major impact on the treatment of Type II diabetes. Since its introduction in the latter part of 1994, it has become a widely prescribed oral hypoglycemic agent. This drug belongs to the class of chemicals called biguanides and has a totally different mechanism of action than the sulfonylureas.

Rather than stimulating the production of insulin in the diabetic who may already have high insulin levels as well as insulin receptors on the cells that do not function normally, this medication *sensitizes the body's cells to insulin's effects*. Thus metformin helps the body utilize its own insulin to process the blood sugar more efficiently. Metformin also inhibits gluconeogenesis (the production of glucose from protein and fat), and reduces the release of glucose from the liver. It facilitates the transportation of sugar across the cell membrane and into the cell where it can be used for energy. *Because it accomplishes this without stimulating insulin secretion, it lowers the blood sugar without the risk of causing hypoglycemia.*

Biguanides were available in the United States in the 1970s as the widely prescribed drug, phenformin. This drug was less effective than metformin and occasionally caused the side effect of lactic acidosis. The occurrence of this serious side effect tarnished the drug's reputation and it was withdrawn from the U.S. market in 1977. Metformin can also cause lactic acidosis, but this can usually be avoided if patients are carefully screened for preexisting kidney or significant liver disease. It should also be avoided by heavy drinkers. Patients undergoing radiocontrast studies such as cardiac catheterization or vascular angiography should be taken off metformin temporarily because of the increased strain that the radioactive dyes place upon the patient's kidneys. Metformin may have some mild side effects. Between 10% and 30% of those taking the medication experience minimal GI symptoms—nausea, vomiting, diarrhea, and anorexia. These symptoms usually subside over time.

Extensive use in Europe has confirmed the benefits and safety of metformin in Type II diabetes when proper screening and monitoring measures are employed.

Some patients with Type II diabetes have a deficiency somewhat analogous to that of Type I diabetes. In these patients, metformin, either alone or in combination with the sulfonylurea drugs, has often proven to be quite effective in achieving glucose control. Metformin potentiates the effects of sulfonylureas.

Studies have shown that metformin has a favorable effect on blood lipids and body weight, which is generally stabilized or decreased.

Thiazolidinediones

Generic name	*Trade Name*
Troglitazone	Rezulin

Note: For patients not responding adequately, Rezulin should be increased at 2 to 4 weeks to 400 mg daily. Maximum dose is 600 mg daily.

Indicated for use in insulin-treated Type II diabetes patients inadequately controlled (Hb1AC>8.5%) with insulin despite over 30 units per day in multiple injections. Rezulin should not be used in Type I diabetes or for the treatment of diabetic ketoacidosis.

Daily Dosage and Titration Guidelines:
Take with a meal. Initial dose: 200 mg; usual dose: 400 mg.

The current insulin dose should be continued upon initiation of Rezulin therapy. It is recommended that the insulin dose be decreased by 10% to 25% when fasting plasma glucose levels decrease to less than 120 mg/dl in patients receiving concomitant insulin and Rezulin. Further adjustments should be individualized based on individual glucose-lowering response.

Rezulin is well tolerated in many different types of patients:

- No differences in effectiveness and safety between patients 65 and over and younger patients.
- No dose ajdustments in patients with renal disease.
- There are no known interactions between Rezulin and laboratory tests.
- Rezulin should be used with caution in patients with liver disease.
- In premenopausal anovulatory patients with insulin resistance, Rezulin treatment may result in resumption of ovulation. These patients may be at risk for pregnancy.
- Rezulin has not been tested in patients with New York Heart Association (NYHA) Class III and IV cardiac status; therefore, caution is advised in administering Rezulin to these patients.
- Safety and effectiveness in pediatric patients have not been established.

Hypoglycemia has not been observed during the administration of Rezulin as monotherapy.

- Patients receiving Rezulin in combination with insulin may be at risk for hypoglycemia and a reduction in the dose of insulin may be necessary.

Drug Interactions
- Cholestyramine reduces the absorption of troglitazone by approximately 70%; thus, coadministration of cholestyramine and Rezulin is not recommended.

Alpha-Glucosidase Inhibitors

Generic name	*Trade Name*
Acarbose	Precose

Initial Dosage—Taken with the first bite of each main meal:
25 mg *tid* (half of a scored 50 mg tablet *tid*)
Alternate Initial Dosage to Minimize GI Side Effects:
25 mg once daily (taken with the first bite of the main meal)
Gradually titrate to: 25 mg *tid*

Titrate to: 50 mg *tid*

Maintenance dosage: 50 mg *tid* to 100 mg *tid*

Maximum dosages: 50 mg *tid* for patients ≤ 132 lbs
100 mg *tid* for patients > 132 lbs

Note: *tid*=three times daily

Acarbose has a unique nonsystemic mode of action. It may be used alone or with a sulfonylurea. The majority of side effects were GI in nature (abdominal pain, diarrhea, and flatulence), which are related to its mode of action—delayed absorption of carbohydrates as a result of competitive inhibition of digestive enzymes. Generally, side effects diminished after 4 to 8 weeks due to adaptation of small intestine enzyme action.

Precose is contraindicated in patients with diabetic ketoacidosis, cirrhosis, colonic ulceration, or partial intestinal obstruction. Because efficacy is similar across dosages greater than 100 mg daily, dosages greater than 100 mg three times a day may be associated with an increased risk of elevation of liver enzyme levels. Dosages greater than 100 mg three times a day are not recommended.

Whether one is taking an oral hypoglycemic agent or not, intelligent management of diabetes remains the same: proper diet, exercise, avoidance of obesity, good hygiene, and a healthy outlook remain the cornerstones of treatment.

11

Patterns of Control and Sick Day Care

- Information Gleaned From Careful Records in Diary Form
- Case Histories
- Sick Day Rules

Although diabetes cannot be cured, it can be controlled. The goal of a control program is to keep blood glucose levels as close to "normal" as possible.

If control is achieved, the person with diabetes will not only feel better about himself, but also will gain better control of the diabetes, rather than the diabetes controlling the person. Also, it is hoped that good control will reduce the risk for future diabetes complications.

Control is achieved by balancing a number of things in your life. You need to balance food intake with energy expenditure (exercise/activity) and with medication (if you are on insulin or oral agents). Your body and your diabetes needs change as you grow older, as your lifestyle changes, and even as you face a new activity, such as a vacation. The balance of your diabetes control plan is upset by these changes and you need to make adjustments in food, exercise, and sometimes medication.

Control is not absolute, nor is it perfect. No one, not even the most experienced diabetes expert, can achieve perfect control of blood glucose. There will be times when some blood glucose levels are high or low. What you want to do is to be as close to good control as possible, most of the time. What you also want to do is know when the *pattern* of blood glucose is above or below normal for a period of time. And you want to be able to find, if possible, what causes these high or low glucose levels, so you can take action to reduce or get rid of the causes.

For you to practice *pattern* control, you need some basic tools:

- You need a diary in which you can record glucose measurements, exercise, food intake, medication, feelings, and events.
- You need a method of measuring glucose:
  1. blood glucose monitoring meter
  2. glucose test strips
  3. Ketone test strips

You need instructions from your physician and diabetic educator on how and when to make adjustments in food, medications, and exercise, based on glucose measurements.

You need to practice *pattern* control on an ongoing basis—day by day, month by month. You will need to do regular, frequent glucose monitoring to develop information about your glucose level patterns. A single, once-a-week glucose test won't give you much information about how your glucose levels have been changing during the previous seven days. A *single* test doesn't show you a pattern, either.

When you make adjustments based on analysis of patterns, you need to be patient and realistic about the results you expect. Sometimes you can get back in good control immediately, but sometimes it may take quite a while.

HOW TO DO PATTERN CONTROL

Monitor your glucose frequently and regularly. Your monitoring schedule should be set when you discuss your management plan with your doctor or educator.

Record all test results in your diary. Take care to record these results accurately.

Write down information about food, exercise, medication, and feelings.

Check your diary every day. If you have a very high or a very low reading, repeat the result and if there is no change, call your doctor or educator.

Review the diary every three to four days. Note if there is a pattern of very high or very low sugar levels for the same time every day.

- Match the time with other factors such as mealtime, exercise, medications, or special events.
- Determine if something out of the ordinary occurred at these times, such as illness or severe stress.

To be effective, pattern control requires you to record as much information as possible in your diary and record it as accurately as you can.

Observations of this type will aid your physician in making appropriate changes in your regimen.

HOW THE PATTERN CONTROL WORKS

Let's suppose that your blood glucose two hours after the noon-time meal for the past three days has been over 200 mg/dl. In the past, it has rarely gone over 175 mg/dl in the afternoon. Your review of the *pattern* in your diary indicates that something is amiss in your control program and you know that you have to do three things to bring your blood glucose levels down into your normal range. You have choices:

- Reduce the quantity of food for your lunchtime meal.
- Increase the time you spend on your after-lunch walking session.
- Increase (with your doctor's permission) the dose of antidiabetic medication.

Remember, a single high postmeal glucose measurement may not need to be acted upon. However, a *pattern* of high, postmeal measurements requires changes in your management program.

Whether you adjust food, medication, or exercise (or a combination of these) should be decided when you discuss your program with your doctor.

Another example of pattern control: Let's suppose that your before-dinner blood glucose readings are in the 50–90 mg/dl range. Your review of the diary shows that you were eating the same meals and injecting the same amount of insulin each day. However, you see in your diary that on Monday, Wednesday, and Friday you participated in a new aerobic exercise program.

That *pattern* of low glucose readings seemed to be linked to your new exercise program. Clearly, something needs to be done to adjust to this beneficial activity without causing an insulin reaction.

Your physician may respond by recommending a larger midday meal, rather than changing the insulin dosage. Or, he may recommend a fruit or cheese snack before your exercise. (Carrying a candy or fruit-juice "emergency" snack with you when exercising can help prevent a hypoglycemic reaction. See Chapter 9.)

ANOTHER EXAMPLE OF PATTERN CONTROL

If the "before breakfast" glucose changes from normal to low, that is a signal that you need to:

- Eat a bedtime snack or change the contents of your nighttime snack.
- Change the evening insulin dosage (with your doctor's supervision).

Remember, a single low blood sugar determination may not be significant, but a pattern of low blood sugars is a clue that changes have to be made.

CASE HISTORIES

Presented here are three case histories that show how *pattern* control can improve management of diabetes.

James Jones

James Jones is a 55-year-old advertising executive who has had Type II (non-insulin-dependent diabetes—NIDDM) for ten years. He is 15 pounds overweight but has managed to control his diabetes by following a meal plan and exercising at a health club three to four times a week. Until recently his predinner sugar levels have stayed between 120 and 150 mg/dl. The past week, however, the glucose levels have risen to 250–300 mg/dl. His diary did not reveal any difference in his meal patterns nor change in his exercise programs. He did note that he had been assigned an important role in his office that meant a great deal to his future financial status.

His doctor recognized that this intense stress was contributing to his lack of good glucose control.

When this was discussed with Mr. Jones, he relaxed and was able to lower his blood sugar levels after the addition of a low-dose oral hypoglycemic agent. In addition, he lowered his noon food intake and increased his exercise program. Within days, he had "taken charge" of his diabetes, and blood sugar levels returned to manageable levels.

Naomi Powell

Naomi Powell is a 15-year-old who has had Type I (insulin-dependent diabetes) for three years. She has maintained good control of her diabetes with two insulin injections a day, a three-meal plus one snack meal plan, and a premeal and bedtime blood glucose monitoring schedule.

As a teenager, Naomi's active life gives her plenty of exercise. Her blood glucose levels have stayed within the normal range that was established by her doctor. She confidently entered high school and tried out for the freshman volleyball team. The team practiced five times a week.

Naomi's diary reveals that her pattern of blood glucose levels remained low (55–60 mg/dl) before her evening meals. She also noted occasional episodes of "wooziness" on her way home after volleyball practice. She also noted in her diary that she felt better on weekends and that her blood sugar levels were more normal.

Naomi's doctor confirmed that the vigorous volleyball exercise could drastically lower her blood glucose levels. He recommended Naomi eat a fruit exchange before the volleyball practice and take a lower midday insulin injection. He also advised an increase in her midday meal.

These measures eliminated the hypoglycemic episodes, and her average blood sugar levels before dinner returned to a range of between 115 and 120 mg/dl.

Margie Mellow

Margie Mellow is 73 years old and has had diabetes for 30 years. She has stayed in good control for most of that time by following a healthy diabetic meal plan, continuing with her gardening exercise daily, and taking a half-hour stroll occasionally with her neighbors.

For the past five years, she has taken a one-a-day oral hypoglycemic agent and has been checking her blood sugar by finger-stick four mornings a week. Margie always keeps a diary of her food intake and blood sugars, and she makes sure to record any marked deviation from her usual activities or blood test results. During "holiday times" she noted a rise in her blood sugars and contacted her physician for further advice. In spite of his recommendations, Margie's diabetes control program no longer was working properly and changes were needed. Her doctor again discussed the need to cut down on food intake to lose extra pounds or to increase exercise. But Margie firmly told her doctor that at her age, she was not about to start running around in athletic clothes and that there were not too many pleasures left in her life that could match a tasty meal. Since neither exercise nor food intake adjustments were practical, Margie's doctor increased the dosage of her oral agent to bring her glucose levels under better control. If this didn't work, he advised, she would have to start taking insulin injections.

These case histories illustrate how important it is to maintain a good record of your activities, exercise routines, and blood glucose determinations. With this important information, your doctor or diabetic educator can make adjustments that will keep you on the right pathway for good diabetic control.

SICK DAY RULES

One of the questions commonly asked by diabetics is "How does my diabetic program change during an illness?" The following answers most of the queries that arise during "sick days":

MEALS: Stay on your regular meal plan if at all possible. In addition, drink lots of fluids—$1/2$ cup of calorie-free broth, soda, or water every hour during the time you are awake. If you are unable to eat regular meals, try to drink fluids containing 10 g of carbohydrates *every* hour you are awake. (Drinks with 10 g carbohydrates include $1/2$ cup regular soda, ginger ale, orange juice, or $1/2$ cup of apple juice.)

MEDICATION: If you inject insulin, stay on your regular schedule even if you are unable to follow your regular meal plan. You may have to increase the dosage of insulin during the illness, so check with your doctor in advance to see how much and when to make an adjustment. Measure your blood glucose before making a dosage change to avoid an insulin-induced low blood sugar reaction.

If you are not taking insulin, you should also stay on your oral hypoglycemic pill to control your diabetes. Do not stop your medication even if you must change your food intake. The illness itself may be *raising* your blood sugar. Certain medications given to treat your illness may have an adverse effect on your blood sugar. This must be checked with your physician.

MONITORING: If you inject insulin, monitor your glucose levels every four hours if possible, and test your urine for ketones at intervals to avoid ketoacidosis. Call your doctor immediately if your blood glucose is very high or if you have moderate to large amounts of ketones in the urine. It is important to report vomiting episodes to your physician before dehydration occurs. If your condition worsens and you cannot reach your doctor, you should go to the nearest hospital emergency room for further advice and treatment.

It is important to continue to keep a close record of your status and additional insulin doses until you are feeling better and your glucose returns toward normal.

During an illness, diabetic patients may have gastrointestinal symptoms that may cause loss of appetite, nausea, vomiting, change in bowel habits, and dehydration. This may cause some patients to alter their insulin dosage for fear of low blood sugar and symptoms of hypoglycemia. It is very important *not* to change insulin or oral medications without specific advice from your doctor or diabetic educator. The reason for this is that the illness itself may be contributing to stress, causing elevation of blood glucose.

It is equally important to take enough food in the form of carbohydrate (starch or sugar) to maintain nutrition and offset any possibility of a hypoglycemic reaction caused by your usual insulin dosage regimen.

The following list of foods can substitute for each serving of starch, milk, or fruit that continue to be necessary during illnesses that have adverse effects on the gastrointestinal system:

$1/2$ cup of hot cereal or 1 slice of bread or toast
1 cup of plain yogurt or $1/2$ cup of ice cream
1 cup of clear soup or $1/2$ cup of egg nog
6 saltine crackers or $1/3$ cup of tapioca

$^1/_3$ cup of fruit juice such as grape, apple, or cranberry juice
2 teaspoons of honey or $2^1/_2$ teaspoons of sugar in a
suitable liquid
$^3/_4$ cup of a cola drink (nondiet) or $^1/_3$ regular Jell-O

Remember that many medications can affect the blood
sugar level. However, your doctor has a wide variety of
drugs that can bring you comfort and relief without
causing marked changes in your diabetic status.

By observing these simple rules and keeping in close
touch with your physician, you can maintain good control of your diabetes even in the face of unpleasant and
debilitating illnesses.

12

Intensive Management of Diabetes

- Effect on Vision
- Renal Function
- Nerve Tissue
- Cardiovascular Disease

The Diabetes Control and Complications Trial (DCCT) is a clinical study conducted from 1983 to 1993 by the National Institute of Diabetes and Digestive and Kidney Diseases (NIDDK). The study showed that keeping blood sugar levels as close to normal as possible slows the onset and progression of eye, kidney, and nerve diseases caused by diabetes. In fact, it demonstrated that *any* sustained lowering of blood sugar helps, even if the person has a history of poor control.

The largest, most comprehensive diabetes study ever conducted, the DCCT involved 1,441 volunteers with insulin-dependent diabetes mellitus (IDDM) and 29 medical centers in the United States and Canada. Volunteers were to have had diabetes for at least one year but no longer than 15 years. They also were required to have no, or only early signs of, diabetic eye disease.

The study compared the effects of two treatment regimens—standard therapy and intensive control—on the complications of diabetes.

Volunteers were divided into two groups:
1. The Primary Prevention Group—Diabetes of short duration (1–5 years) and with absolutely no complications of diabetes.
2. Secondary Intervention Group—These patients demonstrated some early signs of complications such as retinopathy or nephropathy.

The treatment within these two groups was randomized, with some receiving conventional treatment and others receiving intensive management.

The clinical goal for the first group was to attempt to eliminate all symptoms referable to either hyperglycemia or hypoglycemia but not to attempt specific levels of glucose in the blood. The protocol called for three or more insulin injections daily or the use of the insulin pump. (See Chapter 13, *The Insulin Pump.*) Blood was monitored at least four times daily.

Hemoglobin A1c values were determined every three months. Women becoming pregnant in the study were immediately switched to intensive therapy because of the higher incidence of maternal complications of pregnancy and possible congenital malformations of the fetus on conventional treatment.

Intensive therapy included not only dietary control and frequent visits to the clinic, but had as its main goal the maintenance of blood glucose as close to normal as possible: between 70 and 120 mg/dl before meals; under 180 mg/dl after meals; and above 65 mg/dl at 3:00 A.M. to avoid hypoglycemia. Attempts were made to keep the HbA1c below 6.1%. The patients were instructed to monitor blood glucose by finger-stick method four times daily.

The subjects were seen monthly in the participating clinics. Ninety-nine percent were followed for as long as six and a half to eight years.

How Did Intensive Treatment Affect
Diabetic Eye Treatment?

All DCCT participants were monitored for diabetic
retinopathy, an eye disease that affects the retina.

The retina is the light-sensing tissue at the back of
the eye. According to the National Eye Institute, one of
the National Institutes of Health, as many as 24,000 persons with diabetes lose their sight each year. In the
United States, diabetic retinopathy is the leading cause of
blindness in adults under age 65. (See Chapter 17, *Long-
Term Complications of Diabetes.*)

Eye photographs were taken every six months to determine presence or absence of retinopathy. Fifteen percent
of the intensive managed care patients sustained retinopathy while 50% of those subjects under conventional
therapy were found to have retinopathy.

These differences were not observed for the first three
or four years; but after six to eight years the marked
difference in retinopathy between the two groups was
clearly demonstrated.

In Group II, the secondary intervention group, of those
patients who had had some degree of retinopathy at the
beginning of the study, 25% experienced progression of
the retinal lesions, compared to more than 50% in those
treated by conventional therapy.

The study showed marked reduction in risk of retinopathy in both groups of patients who were maintained on
intensive therapy regimes.

How Did Intensive Treatment Affect
Diabetic Kidney Disease?

Participants in the DCCT were tested to assess the
development of diabetic kidney disease (nephropathy).

Findings showed that intensive treatment prevented the development and slowed the progression of diabetic kidney disease by 50%.

Diabetic kidney disease is the most common cause of kidney failure in the United States and the greatest threat to life in adults with IDDM. After having diabetes for 15 years, one-third of people with IDDM develop kidney disease. Diabetes damages the small blood vessels in the kidneys, impairing their ability to filter impurities from blood for excretion in the urine. Persons with severe kidney damage may require a kidney transplant or rely on dialysis to cleanse their blood.

How Did Intensive Treatment Affect Diabetic Nerve Disease?

Participants in the DCCT were examined to detect the development of nerve damage (diabetic neuropathy). Study results showed the risk of nerve damage was reduced by 60% in persons on intensive treatment.

Diabetic nerve damage can cause pain and loss of feeling in the feet, legs, and fingertips. It can also affect the parts of the nervous system that control blood pressure, heart rate, digestion, and sexual function. Neuropathy is a major contributing factor in foot and leg amputations among people with diabetes.

How Did Intensive Treatment Affect Diabetes-Related Cardiovascular Disease?

DCCT participants were not expected to have many heart-related problems because their average age was only 27 when the study began. Nevertheless, they underwent cardiograms, blood pressure tests, and laboratory tests of blood fat levels to look for signs of cardiovascular disease. The study proved that volunteers on intensive treatment had significantly lower risks of developing high blood cholesterol, a cause of heart disease. The risk was 35% lower in these volunteers, suggesting that intensive treatment can help prevent heart disease.

The average HbA1c for the conventional therapy group was 9.0, compared to 7.0 for the intensive-management subjects.

What are the Risks of Intensive Treatment?

In the DCCT, the most significant side effect of intensive treatment was an increase in the risk for low blood sugar episodes—severe hypoglycemia. Because of this risk, DCCT researchers do not recommend intensive therapy for children under age 13, people with heart disease or advanced complications, older adults, or people with a history of frequent severe hypoglycemia.

Adverse effects of intensive therapy included a rather marked increase in weight in some patients, probably secondary to decreased loss of sugar in the urine because of better control, and also an increase in food intake whenever signs or symptoms of hypoglycemia were experienced. For this reason, intensive management may not be appropriate for people with diabetes who are more than moderately overweight.

The most serious side effect of strict control of blood sugars was the increased frequency of serious hypoglycemic episodes. The data showed a threefold increase in serious hypoglycemic attacks when compared to those patients who remained on conventional treatment.

Hypoglycemia was considered "serious" when one of the following occurred:

1. Loss of consciousness
2. Seizure
3. Confusion requiring assistance from an outside source with immediate institution of carbohydrate or glucagon therapy

The main reasons given for choosing intensive management despite the inconveniences demanded by the regimen are as follows:

1. Marked difficulty in stabilizing blood sugars, causing marked variations in glucose levels, ranging from high to low even after attempts to standardize food intake, exercise, and insulin dosage.
2. A strong desire to lower the risk of kidney, eye, nerve tissue, and cardiovascular complications.
3. An unpredictable lifestyle or occupation that makes it almost impossible to follow the same routine from day to day.

Intensive therapy sets stringent goals such as fasting blood sugar of 70–111 mg/dl, prelunch and presupper values of 70–120 mg/dl and levels of 180 mg/dl one hour after meals. To avoid hypoglycemia, the blood sugar should be over 65 mg/dl around 3:00 A.M. In addition, the goal of keeping the glycohemoglobin levels within near normal range requires constant adherence to the regimen advised by the physician and diabetic educator.

There are various methods of dosing and scheduling insulin that are determined by the philosophy of the individual doctor and the patient's response to different schedules. Administering regular insulin before each meal and an injection of NPH at bedtime has worked well for some patients. An alternative method is to give regular insulin before meals and one daily injection of Ultralente.

A mixture of regular and NPH insulin before breakfast, regular insulin before dinner, and an injection of NPH insulin at bedtime has also worked well for some patients.

The above regimens of insulin dosage do not take into account changes in diet, exercise, stress, and other variables that will upset the predominant regular insulin dose routine.

The need to test the urine for ketones remains important not only with conventional diabetic management, but also on the intensive management program.

If you wish to follow an intensive management regimen, your physician will draw a plan for you that will recommend the insulin dosage to be injected, depending on blood glucose levels. Careful home monitoring records must be kept to aid your physician or diabetic educator to elicit a pattern of behavior and food intake. Their relationship to your blood sugars and glycohemoglobin results will determine variations in insulin and dieting changes.

The diet plans prescribed by your doctor and given to you by a dietitian will be tailored to your particular needs and will take into account your height, weight, daily activity, exercise, and other factors. The U.S. dietary goals recommend a variety of foods daily; maintenance of desirable weight; a diet low in fat, particularly saturated fats and cholesterol, high in vegetables, fruits, and grain products; and use of sugar, salt, and alcohol only in moderation.

The proper use of the insulin pump, the role of exercise, and the intensive management of diabetes in pregnancy are discussed in separate chapters.

When a diabetic patient makes the decision to accept the discipline, skill, and responsibilities of intensive insulin control, either by frequent daily injections of insulin or by using the insulin pump, he is making a decision that will lower the risk of diabetic complications and remove much of the fear and apprehension that often accompany the disease.

To qualify as a candidate for intensive diabetic therapy you must:

1. Be under the care of a medical team that can provide the expertise to evaluate and treat your diabetes with regular follow-up supervision.
2. Be knowledgeable about diet and weight control and have the dedication to follow the meal plan designed to avoid the weight gain that is frequently associated with intensive care.
3. Be willing to test your blood four or more times daily—indefinitely.
4. Be willing to accept the increased risk for hypoglycemic reactions.
5. Learn how to treat—or preferably avoid—hypoglycemic reactions.
6. Become knowledgeable under the guidance of your treatment team about adjusting insulin dosage to accommodate changes in lifestyle activities, including taking three or more insulin injections a day or keeping a subcutaneous plastic tube permanently in place to accept insulin delivery from a pump device.
7. Have the financial means or insurance to cover the added cost this regimen entails.

You are not a candidate for intensive treatment if:

1. You have a heart condition that could be adversely affected by a severe hypoglycemic reaction.
2. You have a history of severe hypoglycemic reactions requiring injection of glucagon or treatment in the hospital emergency room.
3. You are under thirteen years of age.

DCCT researchers estimate that intensive management doubles the cost of managing diabetes because of increased visits to health care professionals and the need for more frequent blood testing at home. However, this cost is offset by the reduction in medical expenses related to long-term complications and by the improved quality of life of people with diabetes.

13

The Insulin Pump

- Advantages Over Conventional Treatment
- Description of Equipment and Maintenance
- Getting Started

The U.S.-backed Diabetes Control and Complications Trial (DCCT) showed a firm link between the poor control of diabetes and the eventual development of chronic and disabling complications, including heart disease, neuropathy, visual loss, and kidney disease. (See Chapter 12, *Intensive Management of Diabetes*.)

Present-day treatment of Type I diabetes includes home glucose monitoring, mixed insulins taken at least two times a day, strict adherence to nutrition, proper hygiene, and adequate exercise.

Patients who cannot achieve "rigid" control with the above measures can avail themselves of the insulin pump, an alternative form of treatment that can mimic more closely the body's normal release of insulin to meet its constantly changing requirements. The pump is ideally suited for those who wish to maintain tight control of their diabetes with an intensive treatment regimen.

The pump offers advantages over multiple daily injections of Regular insulin by allowing some freedom from rigid estimations of food intake, sleep, and exercise schedules. These devices provide a constant infusion of "basal" insulin, and are devised to inject a "bolus" of insulin to match carbohydrate consumption at mealtimes.

121

They also permit an adjustment of insulin dosage immediately in response to finger-stick glucose determinations and offer the optimal regulation of blood sugars presently available.

Settings are based on frequent finger-stick blood glucose determinations. The pump delivers a continuous amount of insulin, at a basal rate of 0.5 to 2 units per hour, simulating the normal around-the-clock secretion of insulin. The patient is able to program a lower basal rate at night when blood glucose levels tend to be lowest, and a higher rate during the three to four hours before breakfast when the blood sugars have a tendency to rise (the "dawn" phenomenon). Pumps come with safety features, such as an alarm that warns the user if the insulin level is low or absent, the batteries are low, or the pump is malfunctioning. To guard against the distinct danger of hypoglycemia if too much insulin is accidentally released by the pump, both models have an automatic shut-off valve.

The most important reason for an insulin-dependent diabetic to "go on the pump" is to prevent or delay the serious long-term complications of diabetes, avoid wide fluctuations in blood sugar, provide flexibility in time and size of meals, and easily compensate for increased levels of physical activities. Those that use the pump believe they are availing themselves of the state-of-the-art technique that closely simulates nature's own way of regulating glucose metabolism. Special instructions are needed for showering, bathing, sleeping, and sexual activity. The patient can be "off the pump" for varying periods of time, provided he takes the necessary precautions and is well-versed in his diabetes management.

Carbohydrate, fat, and protein all have impact on blood sugar levels; however, the effect of fat and protein is delayed. Carbohydrate intake is the major factor raising blood glucose levels. Patients are instructed to program the insulin pump, depending on the amount of carbohydrate consumed, intensity of physical activity, finger-stick blood glucose levels, and usual daily needs.

Two battery-powered infusion pumps: the MiniMed 506 or the Disetronic H-Tron V 100 are currently available. These pumps are worn outside the body, weigh less than four ounces, and are about the size of a calling card. A length of plastic tubing connects the pump (containing a reservoir of insulin) to a fine needleless infusion catheter that remains in place under the skin of the abdomen.

The main advantage of pump therapy is that it allows the patient to achieve a degree of metabolic control that is improbable with conventional therapy. The most reliable index of the efficacy of this form of treatment is the level of glycosylated hemoglobin and other parameters of satisfactory glucose control, such as improvement in blood lipids.

There are special considerations associated with pump therapy that must be acceptable to the patient before he can be considered a serious candidate for this alternative to multiple daily injections of insulin.

The patient must:

1. Have the discipline, skill, and determination to perform finger-stick blood determination testing four or more times a day.
2. Be willing to tolerate the inconvenience of wearing the pump.
3. Accept the burden of making adjustments in the microprocessor of the pump depending on food intake, physical activity, stress, travel, and other unforeseen radical changes in everyday activities.
4. Use conscientious sterile techniques.

5. Have family and peer support.
6. Have the resources for the initial financial outlay to purchase the pump and the ability to achieve the proper education from his doctor or diabetic educator.
7. Be aware that infection of the infusion site, serious enough to require antibiotic medication, may occur periodically. The incidence of this untoward side effect can be reduced by changing the infusion site every two or three days.
8. Realize that malfunctioning or pump failure will stop insulin delivery, causing a rapid rise of blood glucose and the possibility of ketoacidosis.

Patients on the pump have to concern themselves with maintaining batteries, checking the infusion catheters, carrying out meticulous skin care, and staying in close touch with their physician and diabetic educator for changes required for "sick days," emergencies such as unusually high or low blood sugars, and radical alterations in lifestyle.

Even after a substantial investment of money and time with trainers in the use of the pump, there is a moderately high "dropout" rate. Long-term studies have not yet been completed on Type II diabetics to prove the theory that use of the pump can prevent or decrease the risk of long-term complications. However, on a theoretical basis, the fine control afforded by the pump would seem to offer the type of blood glucose control that is required to prevent the destructive effect of elevated blood sugars.

GETTING STARTED

The medical team, especially trained in pump therapy, will begin the pump-diabetic patient on a temporary basal rate, food intake, and insulin reduction rate. Formulae for these are based on height, weight, and lifestyle. After experimentation with the beginning formula provided by the diabetic instructor, the patient calculates how his body is reacting to the prescribed diet, insulin, and exercise regimens. There will be times that the sugar appears out of control, causing frustration and disappointment. If the pump is not functioning correctly, an alarm will sound. Occasionally, the batteries will need to be changed or the tube may be dislodged from its place beneath the skin. A visit to the doctor will help in getting back "on track."

The normal *non-diabetic* eats three meals a day and returns his blood glucose level to normal within three hours. This means that the body is exposed to elevated blood glucose for only nine hours out of twenty-four. Without the meticulous control provided by the pump, the diabetic's postmeal sugars would be "high" at least twelve to fourteen hours a day, contributing over many years to the progressive degenerative changes involving the eyes, kidneys, cardiovascular system, and nerve tissue.

Starches are complex carbohydrates that will raise the blood sugar within a two-hour period after eating. This requires enough insulin to bring the sugar to near normal as rapidly as possible and this can be done with greater facility with the pump. Protein does not impact blood sugar as rapidly as carbohydrates because only about 58% is converted into glucose after digestion and its glucose-raising effect may be prolonged until 4–6 hours after eating.

Only 10% of fat is generally converted into sugar; therefore, larger amounts of fat are required to have any significant effect on blood sugar. Additionally, fat takes as long as 10–12 hours to manifest its effect. Two hours after a complex meal consisting of varying amounts of carbohydrate, protein, and fat, the blood should be checked and a reducing dose of insulin administered via the pump if indicated by the results of the test. The basal rate can also be changed if the blood sugar remains elevated, indicating a rise due to the protein and fat contents of the meal. Patients will learn by practice how much insulin is necessary to maintain blood sugar in the 120 mg/dl level by manipulation of the amounts of insulin delivered by the pump. Blood sugar levels as high as 160 mg/dl can be tolerated without drastic changes in the usual insulin regimen.

The basal rate (the amount of insulin needed per hour to maintain an acceptable blood glucose) can be determined by experimentation and close cooperation with the diabetic educator and physician. Some patients require one unit of insulin for every 10 grams of carbohydrate. Others may need .05 units or 1.5 units. This can only be determined by careful record-keeping and frequent comparisons of food intake and insulin requirements. One cannot expect 100% accuracy by this method; therefore, constant guidance by your instructor is mandatory. The ideal formula for obtaining the correct balance of food and insulin while on the pump demands understanding of the individual's carbohydrate/insulin ratio and steady and deliberate dietary planning and exercise routines. If these vary to any great extent, the change in insulin dosage and blood glucose will become apparent within a short period of time.

Once you have estimated your basal rate and required boluses of insulin before meals, you may dispense with some of the finger-stick tests. It is important to rotate sites of finger-stick pricking to avoid sore fingers.

There are many patients who have mastered the use of the pump who agree with their diabetologist that they have achieved the reward of optimal diabetic control as well as a more flexible lifestyle, giving them confidence and satisfaction that the special demands of living with the pump are well worth the effort.

14

Obesity and the Diabetic

- Importance of Weight Control
- Practical Methods of Treatment
- Dietary and Exercise Approach

The vast majority of diabetics have non-insulin-dependent or Type II diabetes (85–90%). The relationship of obesity to Type II diabetes has been clearly established. Medical research has also shown that the susceptibility to disease and early mortality is considerably higher among those who are significantly overweight. *An amazing fact is that weight reduction would allow 75% of Type II diabetics to discontinue their hypoglycemic medications and would lower the blood pressure of most hypertensives.*

Obesity is a common disorder of metabolism that has been recorded from prehistoric times and depicted in ancient sculpture. Obesity may be defined simply as an excess accumulation of fatty tissue. The exact physical criteria of obesity, however, are not clear because variations exist between different cultures, ethnic groups, and even historic time frames. In Western nations, and particularly in the United States, the idealized image for both men and women includes a slender appearance. This concept has been abetted by the fashion world with the aid of the American diet market, that has recorded over 30 billion dollars in gross sales. This figure includes weight-loss programs, health spas, low-calorie foods and soft drinks, weight loss clinics, resort spas, diet books, and appetite suppressants.

Unfortunately, the results of this tremendous expenditure have not slowed the increased incidence of both obesity and diabetes. Twenty-five to thirty-five percent of the American population is considered significantly overweight by the currently accepted standards of measurement.

Significant obesity is usually defined as 20% above the upper normal limit of the theoretical ideal weight as given on the generally accepted actuarial weight charts. The exception to this rule is the heavily muscled individual who will weigh more than the theoretical norm because muscle mass is more dense than adipose tissue.

The majority of obese individuals give a history of being slender until the age of 20–25 years, when noticeable weight gain begins. Progressive weight gain at an approximate amount of five to ten pounds per year continues in those who are destined to become obese.

The public has been barraged with many diverse dietary regimens that include the following:

1. Low protein, high carbohydrate, low fat.
2. High protein, low carbohydrate, high fat.
3. Low protein, low fat, low carbohydrate.

It is no wonder there is confusion regarding weight-loss regimens. Because there are only three different types of foodstuffs, all diets are a result of various combinations of proteins, carbohydrates, and fats. High-fiber content in the diet is beneficial because it adds bulk and the advantage of requiring a longer time to be chewed, thus prolonging the meal. Additionally, the fiber may contribute to the sense of satiety without adding calories to the diet by retaining water and producing a sense of fullness. Many people complain that high-fiber diets are bland and tasteless. Dieters can learn to prepare palatable high-fiber meals from their dietitian or from any of the many high-fiber cookbooks readily available in bookstores.

Formula diets depend on limited quantities of nutrients, often in the form of canned liquids which are designed to contain adequate amounts of protein, minerals, and vitamins. These types of diets are probably most useful when the formula is substituted for breakfast and lunch in conjunction with one low-calorie evening meal. Many patients need the rigidity and discipline of a specific restricted diet plan for long-term success.

A whole spectrum of weight-control advice is offered in newspaper articles, television commercials, and magazines promoting new "healthy" or "miracle" diets. The majority of miracle fad diets are dangerous and lack any scientific justification for their claims. These diets often do not provide essential nutrients, a factor that their proponents often fail to disclose to the consumer. Anecdotal testimonials from those who have used the currently popular weight-control programs are of no significance. Advice offered in the plethora of popular diet books often leaves the reader with confusing counsel on the best methods of losing weight. Even diets that are unsound physiologically often enjoy great popularity and do not lack enthusiastic supporters ready to proclaim their virtues.

Which method really works? Over the short term, results may be achieved with almost any approach that focuses attention on diet and exercise, particularly in a group setting where peer pressure and encouragement from an advisor help to motivate the individual to restrict caloric intake. However, the only success that counts is long-term success.

Many diets, particularly those that cause a rapid weight loss, achieve their dramatic initial results because of water loss. For every gram of stored glycogen or protein that is hydrolyzed for energy, three grams of water are released. This explains the initial "success" of many of the commercial weight loss programs. Two thirds of this weight loss is water, not fat. Following prolonged dieting, physical changes occur in the body that promote sodium and fluid retention. When caloric intake is again increased, rehydration occurs with a rapid weight gain. It is common for female patients, in particular, to "demand" diuretics to correct their swelling and to get rid of their excess retained water. Unfortunately, diuretics can make the problem worse and should not be used to rectify this temporary physiologic phenomenon.

Chronic use of low-calorie diets may actually lead to bingeing. Severe calorie-restriction diets should never be recommended unless there is some medical emergency such as markedly impaired cardiopulmonary function, poorly controlled diabetes, poorly controlled high blood pressure, and perhaps sleep apnea. *A general rule for safe dieting is to not restrict caloric intake below 10 cal per pound of body weight a day.*

The body is a machine. If we ingest more calories than we expend, the excess is converted into fat and stored. If we use more calories than we ingest, the deficit is supplied from our fat reserves and we lose weight. To lose one pound per week requires a decreased caloric intake of 500 calories per day or 3,500 calories per week.

In short, obesity is caused by taking in too many calories, not expending enough energy to burn up the caloric content of the diet that exceeds the body's requirements, or a combination of both of these factors. Additional elements that are more obscure, but that have been shown to play important roles in obesity are:

1. Genetic alterations in the "appetite control center" in the hypothalamic area of the brain that functions as a sort of satiety thermostat.

2. The level of fat in the diet itself. Weight loss is facilitated by diets low in fat even though the caloric intake may be the same as a comparable diet with higher fat content. Over the past eighty years the typical American diet has contained decreased amounts of complex carbohydrates and increased amounts of fat. This is a result of changes in lifestyle which have turned away from nutritious simple home meals high in complex carbohydrates, to high-caloric, high-fat, often prepackaged, or "fast food" items.

3. Eating patterns can contribute to obesity. Skipping breakfast and consuming most of the daily calories with the evening meal can lead to weight gain. People who skip meals burn fewer calories than those who divide their portions into three separate meals.

4. Chronic dieting! Chronic dieting has been shown to lead to a reduction in basal metabolic rate. Chronically dieting people have basal metabolic rates 10–20% below normal. Additionally, because the metabolic rate and caloric needs decline with weight loss, the task of shedding weight becomes more difficult the longer one is on a diet. When the patient resumes a normal diet, weight gain actually occurs more easily than before.

5. Obesity itself. Obese people tend to be less active than nonobese. If caloric intake remains unchanged, increased activity or exercise is the only way to lose weight. Modest increases in physical activity seem to suppress appetite. However, marked increases of physical activity seem to stimulate appetite and caloric intake, although usually not to the extent of the additional calories expended.

Data from the National Health and Nutrition Examination Survey substantiate the claim of many obese people who insist they do not eat more than their lean counterparts. The results showed an inverse relationship between body mass index and mean caloric intake.

6. Abnormalities in the "automatic nervous system" that controls the utilization (burning) of energy.

7. Aging and accompanying inactivity. Basal metabolic caloric requirements gradually decrease with age, although appetite remains unchanged. A continued unchanged caloric intake without the physical activity and exercise required to burn this excess fuel tips the balance toward obesity.

8. Leptin, a newly discovered hormone that has shown remarkable effects on hereditary obesity in laboratory animals. The genetic transmissibility of obesity has been localized on a gene, chromosome 6, in mice. This hormone was isolated from mice that were perpetually overweight.

Leptin acts by decreasing appetite and thereby decreasing food intake. It has also been shown to increase physical activity and causes the animal to "burn" more calories for energy.

It is felt that this hormone acts through the *appetite* or *satiety center* in the hypothalamus of the brain.

Human leptin has been identified and the role of this hormone in relation to human obesity and diabetes is the focal point of investigation and research at the present time.

As discussed in previous chapters, in diabetes there are fewer insulin receptors on muscle, liver, and adipose tissue cell surfaces, thereby contributing to insulin resistance and impaired glucose utilization. After successful weight reduction, there is marked improvement in glucose tolerance and, in many cases of Type II diabetes, the blood glucose levels of sugar will return to normal values.

In addition, the following physiologic consequences occur with higher incidence in overweight persons:

1. Decreased respiratory function and sleep apnea.
2. Increase in high blood pressure, hardening of the arteries, varicose veins, and blood clots in the deep veins of the lower extremities.
3. Gall stones.
4. Strokes.
5. Osteoarthritis and gout.
6. Hyperlipidemia.
7. Increased risk of colon and uterine cancer.
8. Decreased longevity.

Unless the reader understands the basic physiology of nutrition, he will be unable to make an informed judgment of the many different dietary management programs disseminated by books and magazines.

Carbohydrates come in two forms: simple carbohydrates, such as sugar, and complex carbohydrates (fruits, vegetables, and grains).

All carbohydrates consist of combinations of fructose and/or glucose molecules. The simple carbohydrates are called short-chain molecules. The complex carbohydrates, such as wheat bread or spaghetti, are long chains of fructose and glucose.

Complex carbohydrates must be broken down to simple sugar by enzymes in the gastrointestinal tract before they can be utilized for energy or storage for later use. A portion of carbohydrate goes to the liver and is stored as glycogen. The remainder is converted to fat and stored in fatty tissue for later use.

Simple carbohydrates (candy, for instance) are rapidly absorbed into the bloodstream, causing a brisk rise in blood sugar. This rapid rise is often followed by a dip in the blood-sugar level, causing a return of the feeling of hunger. With diabetes, the rise in blood sugar is sustained.

The complex carbohydrates take a longer time to break down into simple sugars and therefore enter the bloodstream at a slower rate with less impact on the blood glucose.

Proteins are the building blocks of all the organs and muscles of the body and are complex molecules made up of long chains of amino acids. Dietary proteins must be broken down to their amino-acid constituents by enzymes before they can enter the bloodstream. Amino acids are essential raw materials needed for the repair, maintenance, and growth of body tissues. Excess amino acids can be converted into glucose for fuel or converted into fat for storage. Nitrogen is produced by these conversions and is excreted by healthy kidneys. If there is renal disease or insufficiency, the buildup of nitrogen products in the blood from protein metabolism may cause a serious medical condition called uremia.

Fat is important for normal metabolism and survival. Fat plays important roles in insulating tissues and supporting the internal organs of the body. Fat is also needed in the outer membranes of cells. Fat is stored in the body in an efficient manner, making it easy to accumulate and difficult to remove except by reducing caloric intake below body requirements. Fat supplies nine calories per gram, whereas carbohydrate and protein provide only four calories per gram. Most tissues will use or prefer to use carbohydrate to provide their energy needs. The brain, however, relies exclusively on carbohydrates for its metabolic processes.

The diabetic diet is simply a well-balanced diet that

meets the nutritional needs of the diabetic and everyone else. The standard ADA diabetic diet has been modified in recent years by reducing the fat content and increasing the fiber content as research has shown the benefits of these changes for everyone.

To achieve long-term weight loss requires a change in dietary habits with the advice and guidance of a trained dietitian combined with long-term follow-up. Eating habits and behavioral characteristics have to be altered and maintained in conjunction with a well-planned exercise regimen. Obesity is a chronic disease and needs long-term support and guidance to be treated successfully.

Pharmacologic approaches to treating obesity include amphetamines. These drugs have undesirable side effects including elevation of blood pressure, a rapid heart rate, nervousness, sweating, anxiety, and a marked propensity to cause addiction. These medications are no longer recommended nor are they approved by the FDA for the treatment of obesity.

Phenylpropanolamine and ephedrine are the only over-the-counter obesity drugs currently available. These drugs are only minimally effective as anorectics and carry the risk of elevation of blood pressure and increasing the chance for a stroke.

Orlistat is the first of a new class of non-systemic anti-obesity drugs called lipase inhibitors, or fat blockers, which act in the gastrointestinal tract to prevent the absorption of fat by about 30%. Drugs in this class are not absorbed from the intestinal tract and therefore do not achieve their effect through changes in brain chemistry or other systemic reactions. The drug will be marketed under the trade name Xenical.

According to the data from a large study with the drug, almost three times as many patients on Xenical with a moderately reduced caloric diet lost 10% or more of body weight compared to placebo with diet. Nearly twice as many patients on Xenical lost at least 5% of body weight compared to placebo with diet. The average patient in one-year clinical trials weighed 220 pounds and lost 20 pounds, or about 10% of body weight, after taking Xenical and being on a moderately reduced calorie diet. Many patients who continued into the second year of the studies were able to keep off the lost weight. Long-term studies on Xenical have not yet been completed.

Serotonin is a naturally occurring substance that plays a key role in transmitting messages in the brain. Anorectic drugs that work by altering serotonin activity are called serotonin reuptake inhibitors. Drugs in this class have proven effective, at least in the short term, in promoting weight loss. The two currently popular serotonin reuptake inhibitors are Redux (Desfenfluramine), which is used alone at a dosage of 15 mg twice daily, and Pondamin (Fenfluramine), which is usually taken at a dosage of 20 mg three times daily. In recent times Pondamin has enjoyed widespread popularity when used in combination with Phenteramine, a drug that has pharmacological properties related to the amphetamines. Fastin, Ionamin, and Adipex P are three such drugs whose chief ingredient is Phenteramine. The combination of any of these drugs with Pondamin has come to be known popularly as the "Fen-Phen" regimen. Despite the widespread use and popularity of this combination of anorectics, such use does not have FDA approval.

The Serotonin reuptake inhibitors are recommended only for people with significant obesity—those with a body mass index of 30 or higher, or 27 or higher if there are associated risk factors such as diabetes, high blood pressure, or dyslipidemia. Body mass index is calculated by taking the person's weight in kilograms, divided by his height in meters, then squared. To make the metric conversion weight in pounds, divide by 2.2 = weight in kilograms. Inches multiplied by 0.0254 = meters. The following chart can serve as a quick guide to estimate your body mass index.

BODY MASS INDEX (BMI), kg/m²						
	——— Height (feet, inches) ———					
Wt (lbs)	5'0"	5'3"	5'6"	5'9"	6'0"	6'3"
140	27	25	23	21	19	18
150	29	27	24	22	20	19
160	31	28	26	24	22	20
170	33	30	28	25	23	21
180	35	32	29	27	25	23
190	37	34	31	28	26	24
200	39	36	32	30	27	25
210	41	37	34	31	29	26
220	43	39	36	33	30	28
230	45	41	37	34	31	29
240	47	43	39	36	33	30
250	49	44	40	37	34	31

All appetite suppressant drugs increase the risk of developing primary pulmonary hypertension (PPH), a serious and often fatal disorder. This illness occurs in the general population at a rate estimated to be one or two cases per one million persons yearly. There does not appear to be a significant increase in the incidence of PPH in those who take anorectic drugs for three months or less. However, longer use of appetite suppressants increases the risk to approximately 18 persons per million per year for those taking the anorectic drugs. The longer one stays on appetite suppressants, the greater the danger of this dreaded complication. Admittedly, the incidence of PPH is low, even with the serotonin reuptake inhibitors. However, if you are the one afflicted with PPH, your weight loss program could prove to have been a fatal therapeutic misadventure. It certainly is wise to limit the use of any of the anorectics. Those who choose to go on these drugs must remain on guard against PPH, and report to the physician any signs of its development. The initial symptoms are usually shortness of breath, angina (chest discomfort from coronary artery insufficiency), fainting, and sometimes lower extremity edema (swelling of the legs). Unfortunately, once symptoms become apparent, treatment is not always successful.

The main question to be decided is "Are anorectic drugs effective in the long term for most people?" Obese adults who seek medical help for weight loss, who are given dietary management instruction and anorectic medication, do lose more weight than those treated with placebo and diet, at least in the short-term studies. The difference in weight loss between the drug-treated patients and those receiving placebo and dietary instruction is, however, only minimal and often only a fraction of a pound per week. The rate of weight loss is greatest in most trial studies for both drug- and placebo-treated subjects during the first few weeks and usually decreases in succeeding weeks.

The average weight loss with the various anorectic drugs varies from trial to trial and is undoubtedly influenced by such factors as the specific dietary regimen prescribed, the patient's physician or patient's counselor relationship, and the population group under study. Obesity usually develops gradually over the years. Successful treatment must also be long term and involve changes in eating habits and lifestyle that promote gradual weight loss and adherence to the new regimen to ensure maintenance of the pounds shed.

Before making a serious commitment to a weight-reduction diet and exercise program, you should have a complete medical exam by your physician. He will check your heart and blood pressure and look for any contraindications to your anticipated exercise and dietary regimen. Losing pounds is just the beginning. Be prepared to follow an intelligent approach to nutrition and physical activity that will remain with you for the rest of your life. In the beginning, you will feel satisfaction as your weight declines. If you relapse, you will feel anguish and depression. Be prepared for these mixed emotions. Conquering your obesity and lowering the risk for all the possible medical and surgical events that are associated with it will raise your self-esteem and bring about a "good feeling" that you may not have had for years. There will be no more self-pity, resentment, or guilt feelings in regard to food, and most important, your diabetes will be much easier to control and blood sugar may return to normal.

It is difficult to achieve normal body weight without a great deal of introspection, self-discipline, and reenforcement of your self-esteem. One must realize that obesity is a chronic disease not unlike high blood pressure or diabetes.

Because obesity is a chronic problem, treatment must be continuous. Many people do not understand the necessity for lifelong intensive treatment, and instead seek easy short-term solutions.

Attempting to lose weight with the latest fad diet will not work. Skipping meals and bingeing later will not work. The obese patient must accept an intelligent, nutritious diet plan, adopt a daily exercise routine, and remain on this regimen for the rest of his life. Your health and your appearance will make it all worthwhile.

15

Benefits of Exercise

- Beneficial Effects on Metabolism
- Medical Clearance for Exercise
- Appropriate Exercise Programs

Physical activity has been a part of daily life from the earliest caveman pursuing prey in his search for food or fleeing ferocious animals in his struggle to survive, to such current day chores as shoveling snow or mowing grass.

In today's society, especially in "advanced" western nations like the United States, the general population has become more sedentary, riding in cars to school or work, sitting at desks, and using elevators instead of stairs and vacuum cleaners instead of brooms. And let's not forget the couch potato sitting in front of the television, munching on snacks.

More than 35% of all Americans are significantly overweight. For the Type II diabetic this is disastrous. We have discussed the significant adverse effects of obesity on non-insulin-dependent diabetics (Type II) in Chapter 14, *Obesity and the Diabetic*. The obese may have normal blood insulin levels, but physiologically there is a *relative* lack of insulin because:

1. The larger body mass requires more insulin.
2. There are fewer insulin receptors on body cells for the insulin molecule to attach to and transport glucose

across the cell membrane and into the cell where it can be utilized for energy.

3. There is decreased insulin *binding* to specific receptors on the surface of the cell. (Insulin-receptor binding is 50% lower in the obese diabetic.)

4. There is decreased sensitivity of insulin response to glucose.

We often use the term *resistance* when referring to the above factors in relation to the glucose response to insulin in Type II diabetes and obesity.

While diet and achievement of normal body weight is often considered the therapeutic goal in Type II diabetes, the other equally important half of the equation is exercise and physical training.

Restrictions of caloric intake and increased physical activity have a direct, beneficial effect on cell-receptor affinity and number, i.e., overcoming insulin resistance.

While exercise has benefits for everyone, it is especially important for patients with diabetes. Physical activity of all types, and particularly regular aerobic exercise, helps receptor cells function more efficiently, aids in the utilization of glucose at a more rapid rate, reduces blood lipids (cholesterol, triglycerides), and raises the "good" high-density cholesterol (HDL).

Other benefits of exercise include lowering high blood pressure and slowing the development or reducing the incidence of chronic complications.

Exercise increases the efficiency of the respiratory and cardiovascular systems and improves blood circulation. A daily exercise routine reduces stress and imparts a sense of well-being that many patients feel is important in their everyday activities.

During exercise, there is an increased utilization of

calories. The calories burned vary, depending on the intensity and duration of the activity.

With strenuous exercise, the heart may pump 5 to 6 times its resting output, and the amount of oxygen utilized may increase twentyfold. More than 90% of the "fuel" used during heavy exertion comes from glucose and free fatty acids. The glucose in the bloodstream can be used up in about four minutes of strenuous physical activity. The body then turns to the liver to supply additional energy from the breakdown of glycogen stores. In the non-diabetic, insulin levels rise to meet the demand of this increase in blood glucose. In the diabetic, the deficiency of insulin can cause the blood sugar to fall because there is insufficient insulin to mobilize glucose from stored glycogen. Increasing carbohydrate intake is the most rapid and convenient way to maintain the blood sugar in a satisfactory range during exercise. If the physical activity remains fairly similar from day to day, and finger-stick blood sugars are obtained before and after exercise for several days, the diabetic patient soon finds the correct amount of carbohydrate and insulin dosage to stay well regulated. Diabetics using the pump soon learn how much basal insulin is required, how often a bolus of insulin is needed, and how to set the computerized meter accordingly. For best performance, the blood glucose should be kept between 70 and 150 mg/dl. *Hypoglycemia in this situation always indicates an excessive blood insulin level.* To insure the availability of glucose and fat for conversion to energy, insulin levels in the blood must be accurately regulated.

As noted, physical activity, under the supervision and guidance of your physician, has beneficial effects on the cardiovascular system, lipid levels, kidney function, and emotional status. The aim is to increase muscle strength, improve cardiac and pulmonary function, and, most important, regulate blood sugar and reduce the risk for the complications associated with diabetes.

Before beginning an exercise program, a thorough checkup including a cardiovascular assessment by your doctor is necessary. He will evaluate your physical and medical status and prescribe the proper amount and types of exercise on an individual basis. He will want to examine your heart, eyes, feet, circulation, and kidney function before you start on a rigid regimen of physical activity.

If you have had diabetes for more than seven years, are over 35 years of age, have a family history of heart disease, or are planning a strenuous exercise program, the doctor may recommend a "stress" electrocardiogram. The routine ECG done lying at rest may not reveal important cardiac abnormalities that become apparent only when extra work demands are made of the heart. The "stress" ECG monitors the heart while you run on a treadmill; it may reveal abnormal rhythms or evidence of coronary artery blood flow insufficiency to this vital organ.

Once the doctor's evaluation and recommendations are concluded, you may embark on a proper physical activity program. A daily record of oral hypoglycemic medications or insulin doses should be kept when you commence your exercise program. Select an aerobic activity. Walking, swimming, and bicycling are examples of aerobic activities that do not place undue stress on the joints. Patients with peripheral neuropathy are advised to avoid jogging because they may be insensitive to blisters or cuts that may develop on their feet. Those patients who have retinopathy or nephropathy should avoid jarring activities that can raise the blood pressure, such as weight-lifting or racquetball. If you have not been active, begin your exercise program progressively with five to ten minutes of activity three or four times a week, and work up gradually to sessions of thirty minutes or more. In this manner, you can increase your endurance with minimal risk of injury. Always begin your exercise program with a gradual warm-up period consisting of at least five minutes of stretching or walking normally.

To avoid either a hypoglycemic or hyperglycemic reaction, it is advised that you eat a meal one or two hours before beginning your workout. If you are participating in prolonged strenuous activity such as jogging, tennis, swimming, racquetball, or school athletics, decreasing insulin and/or taking a 15–20 gram carbohydrate snack every half hour to compensate for the additional caloric need, can allow sports participation without undue fear or apprehension.

However, if you develop a headache, feel nervous or shaky, cool and clammy, or weak, STOP exercising immediately and check your blood sugar. If there is a doubt about the status of your glucose level, eat a snack. Exercise may have a prolonged effect on blood sugar, resulting in hypoglycemia for up to twenty-four hours.

Any shortness of breath, tightness, or chest pain radiating down the arm or into the neck or shoulders, that lasts for more than a few seconds, must be regarded seriously as a possible sign of cardiovascular disease requiring prompt medical attention.

Hyperglycemia, accompanied by ketoacidosis, is seen primarily in those with Type I diabetes. If the blood sugar is 240 mg/dl or above, it is recommended that the workout period be abandoned. The urine should then be tested for ketones. Consult your diabetologist; an extra dose of insulin may be in order.

It is important to wear the proper shoes or athletic sneakers to avoid any blisters, corns, or calluses. Walking, running, or jogging can conceivably be associated with thickening of the outer layers of the skin of the feet (hyperkeratosis), giving rise to calluses. Also, perspiration and dirt can be the nidus for blisters or infection, so a thorough examination of the feet should be a part of your exercise routine. Comfortable clothing and an ID bracelet should be carried in a convenient place; and, of course, a readily available quick source of carbohydrate is essential.

Exercise should be done on a regular basis, at least three times a week, at a convenient time; blood glucose levels should be monitored when necessary; a snack should always be available; and shoes and clothing must be selected carefully. (See Chapter 20, *Care of the Feet.*) Remember to replenish water at frequent intervals, depending on the temperature and the activity, and don't forget to warm up and cool down.

In the beginning, glucose monitoring is essential to evaluate minor or major changes resulting from burning additional calories during physical activity.

After strenuous exercise, it is best to slow the pace gradually to let the accelerated physiological responses to exercise slowly return to normal. Spend at least five to ten minutes slowing down. This means moving at approximately 25% of your normal exercise rate. *The slow-down period is equally or perhaps more important than the warm-up period.*

In Type I diabetics, a finger-stick blood sugar test should be done, and by carefully monitoring your food and insulin needs before and after your exercise program, hypoglycemia can be avoided. If the sugar is low, a snack of orange juice or Coca-Cola is necessary to avoid a low sugar reaction.

On rare occasions, vigorous prolonged physical effort can precipitate rises in blood sugar, making it wise to check finger-stick glucose after the event.

In summary, exercise is very important in increasing

strength and endurance, easing emotional tensions, and aiding in weight reduction.

The exercise should be done regularly at a convenient time. Blood glucose levels should be monitored when necessary, and a snack should be readily available.

16

Diabetes, Lipids, and Atherosclerosis

- Definition of "Good" and "Bad" Cholesterol
- Decreasing Risk of Cardiovascular Disease
- Newest Drugs for Treatment

Lipids is the comprehensive term for a group of fat and fatlike substances that play a major role in the development of atherosclerosis (hardening of the arteries). Dyslipidemia (pronounced dis-lip-id-eem-ee-uh) means abnormal levels of lipids in the blood. Diabetics are more prone than non-diabetics to have dyslipidemia. The most common type of dyslipidemia is an abnormally high level of cholesterol and triglycerides, a type of fat that serves as fuel storage for the body.

Although cholesterol has become a household word, much confusion remains regarding this waxy, fatlike substance. Perhaps no other element in our diet has been the source of such intense controversy. However, the jury is no longer out; a verdict has been rendered. Case closed. The Framingham epidemiological study of more than 5,000 men and women over a twenty-five-year period showed a definite link between elevated cholesterol and heart disease. Other risk factors identified were cigarette smoking, sedentary lifestyle, and high blood pressure.

Cholesterol is vital for performing a number of essential biological functions. It is required for building body cells

147

and plays an important role in the synthesis of certain hormones. To meet these needs, "Mother Nature" has provided for the liver to manufacture adequate amounts of cholesterol. Cholesterol is also obtained from certain food products of animal origin. Although cholesterol is found only in products of animal origin, saturated fats, whether derived from animal or vegetable products, are readily converted into cholesterol when they are metabolized by the body. *Saturated fats in the diet play an even greater role than dietary cholesterol in raising blood cholesterol levels.*

"Oil and water don't mix." Body fluids—blood, serum, and lymph—are all water based. Lipids are not soluble in water. For lipids to enter the body fluids and be transported throughout the body they must link up with proteins, forming compounds called lipoproteins. The protein is the transport vehicle and the lipid is the cargo.

There are two significant types of lipoproteins involved in the transport of cholesterol. Low-density lipoproteins (LDL) and high-density lipoproteins (HDL). The LDL (LDL cholesterol) delivers the cholesterol to the body's cells. However, when there is an excess amount of cholesterol the surplus may be deposited on the walls of the blood vessels, forming scarred areas called plaques. Thus begins the atherosclerotic process that can eventually choke and clog the artery. For this reason, LDL is called "bad" cholesterol.

The HDL cholesterol removes excess cholesterol from the blood, and new evidence reveals it sometimes removes it from the plaque deposits as well, carrying it back to the liver, where it can be reused or broken down and excreted. HDL is therefore called "good" cholesterol.

If the LDL cholesterol remains elevated through the years, the lumen or opening of the blood vessel may gradually narrow as the plaque deposits enlarge and encroach on the lumen. When the opening is completely occluded, the tissue beyond the point of occlusion becomes necrotic (dies).

Atherosclerosis is an ongoing dynamic process. Severe lesions that occlude an important vessel certainly pose a major risk. However, the vast majority of vessels that become completely occluded by a thrombus were not blocked for more than 30–50% of their diameter by atheromatous plaques, prior to the thrombosis. To understand this phenomenon, it is necessary to review the changes that give rise to plaque formation.

The body attempts to protect itself from the harmful LDL cholesterol with scavenger cells called macrophages. These watchdog cells ingest the LDL cholesterol and are transformed into what are known as foam cells. The foam cells undergo necrosis and die, discharging their lipid-rich contents into the ever-growing core of the plaque. Thus, the body's attempt to protect itself from the harmful LDL cholesterol in the blood backfires when the LDL-laden macrophages discharge their contents into the wall of the blood vessel, forming plaques. The ever-enlarging plaques are covered by the endothelium—the inner lining of the blood vessels—that forms a thin, unstable covering over the plaque. The ever-growing, lipid-rich plaque pool is like a time bomb waiting to go off. When the weak endothelial cap of the plaque ruptures, the lipid-rich core material is brought into contact with the blood. Because this material is highly thrombogenic (prone to cause a thrombosis), clotting rapidly ensues and the vessel is suddenly clogged.

Before the LDL cholesterol can gain entry into the macrophages, it must be oxidized. Studies have shown that antioxidants can help protect against heart disease by preventing this oxidation from taking place. Vitamin E, at doses of 400 I.U. of D-Alpha Tocopherol, is the recommended daily dose to help inhibit this oxidative process.

Larger doses may have undesirable side effects and are to be avoided. Vitamin C is also a potent antioxidant and many cardiologists recommend 1,000 mg daily as the optimum dose for their patients.

For years the endothelium was considered to be a simple semipermeable membrane. It is now known that the endothelial cells produce vital substances that play key roles in maintaining the normal dilation of the blood vessels. Chief among these is nitric oxide, which it manufactures from the essential amino acid L-Arginine. It is unknown whether oral supplements of this amino acid can help to protect against endothelial damage. However, L-Arginine supplements may have untoward side effects.

The traditional major risk factors for heart disease, high blood pressure, dyslipidemia, and cigarette smoking are all associated with impairment of endothelial function. Modification of these factors, particularly lowering of the LDL cholesterol, improves endothelial function. Cigarettes, another major risk factor for atherosclerosis, cause their damage by impairing endothelial function, promoting oxidation of LDL cholesterol, and causing vasoconstriction that elevates blood pressure as well as increasing platelet agglutination, which is the first step in blood clotting. Research studies have clearly demonstrated that Vitamin C improves endothelial function in smokers. Every smoker would be well advised to take his daily dose of Vitamin C.

For the blood-clotting mechanism to begin, certain particles that normally circulate in the blood, called platelets, are required. The clotting process is initiated when the platelets become sticky and adhere to one another and the blood vessel wall. Ordinary aspirin has the effect of preventing this platelet stickiness from developing. Aspirin, in low doses, has been used to reduce the risk of heart attacks. The dose of aspirin required is small. One baby aspirin or one enteric-coated 80 mg aspirin, equivalent to the baby aspirin tablet, daily suffices. An alternative satisfactory schedule is one whole aspirin or Ecotrin (coated aspirin) every other day.

Despite a declining death rate from many causes, coronary artery disease still ranks as the number one killer in America. This is particularly true not only for those over the age of 65, but also for men in the 45–65 year-old age group. As one would suspect, middle-aged men with coronary artery disease are generally found to have significantly higher levels of cholesterol and triglycerides than those without heart disease.

It has long been known that diabetics are prone to developing atherosclerosis and heart disease about ten to twelve years earlier than the population at large. The dyslipidemia with elevated cholesterol and triglycerides associated with diabetes correlates directly with the accelerated vascular aging associated with the disease. Coronary disease is now the chief cause of death in diabetics, and the incidence is rising. In Type I diabetes, cardiovascular abnormalities are markedly accelerated and may appear in the 20–30 year-old age group. Before the discovery of insulin, most diabetics died from ketoacidosis, a direct metabolic complication of their disease. Diabetics can now live fairly normal lives, but there is still the specter of accelerated vascular disease. Controlling blood sugar, along with lowering blood cholesterol and triglycerides, significantly reduces the risk of developing atherosclerosis and heart disease. Management of elevated lipids along with avoidance of other risk factors such as smoking, the maintenance of normal blood pressure, and getting adequate exercise, markedly reduce the risk of heart disease in the diabetic patient.

CHOLESTROL LEVEL GUIDELINES

The medical guidelines for classifying blood cholesterol levels advise that a total cholesterol level of less than 200 mg/dl is "desirable" for adults. There are three categories of total cholesterol:

Total Cholesterol Categories:

Desirable Blood Cholesterol	Borderline-High Blood Cholesterol	High Blood Cholesterol
less than 200 mg/dl	200–239 mg/dl	240 mg/dl and above

Cholesterol levels less than 200 mg/dl are considered desirable, while levels of 240 mg/dl or above are high and require more specific attention. Levels from 200–239 mg/dl also require attention, especially if the HDL cholesterol is low or LDL level is high or if there are two or more other risk factors for heart disease.

LDL Cholesterol

Desirable	Borderline-High Risk	High Risk
less than 130 mg/dl	130–159 mg/dl	above 160 mg/dl

The LDL level gives a better picture of the risk for heart disease than the total cholesterol level. Accordingly, most physicians consider lowering LDL as the main treatment goal for a cholesterol problem. If your LDL level puts you at high risk and you have fewer than two other risk factors for heart disease, your target goal should be an LDL level of less than 160 mg/dl. However, if you have two or more other risk factors for heart disease, your LDL goal should be less than 130 mg/dl. If you already have heart disease, your LDL target should be even lower—100 mg/dl or less. These target goals suggested by the National Cholesterol Educational Program (NCEP), may be summarized as follows:

HDL CHOLESTEROL

Normal HDL	Low HDL	High HDL
more than 35 mg/dl	less than 35 mg/dl	above 60 mg/dl

Unlike total cholesterol and LDL cholesterol, the lower your HDL, the higher your risk for heart disease. An HDL level less than 35 mg/dl is considered low and increases your risk for heart disease. The higher your HDL, the better. An HDL level of 60 mg/dl or above is high and is associated with longevity. Alcohol raises the HDL. However, the chemical fraction of the HDL elevated by alcohol is not the portion of HDL cholesterol that is protective against atherosclerosis. Therefore, high HDL levels in alcoholics can give a distorted view of the significance of this finding. An HDL level below 35 is considered a risk factor. An HDL over 60 usually is protective—a negative risk factor. HDL levels are particularly effective in their protective action in females. It is therefore probably fair to place more weight on the significance of levels of HDL cholesterol in women than in men.

Your doctor should look at all your risk factors to decide what measures to take to lower your blood cholesterol and reduce your risk of heart disease.

CHOLESTEROL/HDL RATIO

The importance of the level of total cholesterol can be determined only after evaluation of the types of cholesterol that contribute to the total reading. A frequently simplified formula that yields practical information is the ratio of total cholesterol to HDL cholesterol.

A total cholesterol level of 260 mg% may have entirely different significance for two individuals with different lipid metabolism. If the HDL level is high, the ratio may be within normal limits and not represent a health threat despite the high total cholesterol level. If the HDL were low, the elevated cholesterol would require management. Even though the general guidelines state that a cholesterol level below 200 mg% is desirable, if an individual with a low cholesterol reading has a low HDL level, the ratio would be high and indicate vulnerability to cardiovascular disease. Conversely, as noted, an individual with a high total cholesterol, with a high HDL cholesterol, might well have a satisfactory total cholesterol/HDL ratio and not be at risk for cardiovascular disease. The following reference values can serve as a general guide:

Coronary Heart Disease Risk*	_Total Cholesterol/HDL Ratio_	
	Male	Female
$1/2$ Average	3.4	3.3
Average (normal)	5.0	4.4
Twice Average (moderate)	9.6	7.0
Three Times Average (high)	13.4	11.0

*Data based on Farmingham Study

TRIGLYCERIDES

Triglycerides are fats that circulate in the blood and serve as energy sources. Based on your age, your triglyceride levels should not rise above the following:

AGE	INCREASED RISK
19–29	> 140 mg/dl
30–39	> 150
40–49	> 160
> 49	> 190

Triglyceride levels must be done on blood obtained after an overnight fast of at least 14 hours, otherwise erroneously high levels may result. Total cholesterol levels may be performed on non-fasting blood. HDL cholesterol levels, however, must be done on fasting specimens for accurate results.

RISK FACTORS FOR HEART DISEASE

Factors You Can Do Something About

Cigarette smoking
High blood cholesterol (high total cholesterol and high
   LDL cholesterol)
Low HDL cholesterol
High blood pressure
Diabetes
Obesity/overweight
Physical inactivity

Factors You Cannot Control

Age
   45 years or older for men
   55 years or older for women
Family history of early heart disease (heart attack or
   sudden death)
   Father or brother—stricken before the age of 55
   Mother or sister—stricken before the age of 65

WHAT AFFECTS YOUR
BLOOD CHOLESTEROL LEVEL?

Your blood cholesterol level is affected by:

What you eat—The saturated fat and cholesterol in the food you eat raise total and LDL cholesterol levels.

Overweight—Being overweight can make your LDL cholesterol level go up and your HDL level go down.

Physical activity/Exercise—Increased physical activity helps to lower LDL cholesterol and raise HDL cholesterol levels.

Heredity—Your body makes all the cholesterol it needs, and your genes influence how your body makes and handles cholesterol.

Age and sex—Blood cholesterol levels in both men and women begin to go up at about age 20. Women before menopause have levels that are lower than men of the same age. After menopause, a woman's LDL cholesterol level goes up—and so does her risk for heart disease. This can be countered by the administration of the female hormone, estrogen, but only if your physician feels it is appropriate in your case.

DYSLIPIDEMIA IN DIABETICS

Lowering blood lipids is considered imperative in patients with known coronary artery disease. Because diabetes itself constitutes a significant risk factor for dyslipidemia, diabetics would be well advised to aim for the same target goals set by the NCEP for individuals with known heart disease.

The chain of events that culminates in dyslipidemia with its consequences and sequelae in diabetics begins with elevated insulin and blood sugar levels. As emphasized throughout this book, the main goal of diabetes treatment is to normalize blood sugar, which can be deemed to have been accomplished when the hemoglobin A1c levels are 7% or less.

Type II diabetes is characterized by insulin resistance, increased insulin levels in the blood, and dyslipidemia with the prominent features of elevated LDL cholesterol and triglyceride blood levels, dyslipidemic factors that predispose to atherosclerosis. Macrovascular (large vessel) disease with progression of atherosclerosis in the coronary arteries, cerebral vessels, and peripheral vessels is commonly encountered in Type II diabetes. Microvascular (small vessel) disease, the type that predominates in Type I diabetes, is responsible for retinopathy, neuropathy, and nephropathy. These same microvascular changes are also found with Type II diabetes. In fact, hyperglycemia sufficient to be associated with retinopathy is one of the diagnostic criteria physicians consider when evaluating a patient for Type II diabetes.

The conventional invasive treatments for cardiovascular disease such as coronary artery bypass surgery and angioplasty have not yielded satisfactory results when performed on diabetics. Development of atherosclerosis in the bypass segments is often quite rapid as well as a mortality incidence associated with the procedure that is considerably higher than in non-diabetics. The high five-year mortality rate for Type II diabetics undergoing coronary artery angioplasty is undesirable, although the use of stents to maintain the integrity of the blood vessels has improved the outlook for this procedure.

The high incidence of macrovascular disease in Type II diabetes and the poor results from conventional surgical intervention mandate very aggressive management of dyslipidemia.

Studies have shown that insulin stimulates the production

of triglycerides, which in turn promotes the synthesis of LDL cholesterol. Incidentally, the levels of HDL cholesterol in the blood are inversely proportional to the increased triglyceride levels.

A high complex-carbohydrate, high-fiber, and low-fat diet permits for more efficient utilization of insulin. This type of diet prolongs absorption time because the complex biochemical changes required to break down complex carbohydrates into their simple sugars does not cause an insulin surge as would occur with a diet of refined foods such as white rice, white bread, and foods containing simple sugars.

Diet and regular exercise play critical roles in controlling blood sugar, improving endothelial function, and ameliorating insulin resistance. Physical activity also exerts a beneficial effect by utilizing glucose as the fuel for the energy expended in performing the physical activity, thereby also reducing the demand for insulin.

Hypertension also requires aggressive treatment because elevated blood pressure can play a contributory role in the development of atherosclerosis. Additional benefits of treating high blood pressure are the reduction in the risk for stroke and nephropathy. Beta-blockers, sometimes used to treat high blood pressure, may contribute to elevating LDL levels and lowering HDL levels. Thiazide diuretics may have the undesirable side effect in diabetics of elevating blood sugar. Ace inhibitors can exert a renal protective action and may aid in preventing nephropathy.

Some people are born with defective metabolic pathways for metabolizing the amino acid homocysteine. This defect may predispose to atherosclerosis. It can be detected by a simple (but expensive) blood test. Folic acid supplements at a dosage of 1 mg/day can correct this condition. If your diet does not contain adequate amounts of folic acid, supplementation is advised.

A recently completed long-term study of Western Electric employees on fish diets demonstrated an inverse relationship between the quantity of fish consumed over the years and coronary artery mortality. The protective effect, although unknown, is something other than the Omega 3 fatty acid content of the fish. In fact, dietary supplementation with fish oil capsules is not recommended.

Dyslipidemia that cannot be brought under control by careful management of diabetes, weight reduction, and adequate exercise calls for a search for secondary causes of hyperlipidemia (i.e. hypothyroidism, genetic hypercholesterolemia, kidney or liver disease, alcoholism). If these secondary causes of dyslipidemia are ruled out, drug therapy must be considered by the physician to aid in reducing the blood lipids.

The American Heart Association recommends that the first step in the treatment of elevated cholesterol and LDL is diet. They limit dietary cholesterol to less than 300 mg per day, less than 30% total fat, and less than 10% saturated fat per day. A more aggressive approach to lowering cholesterol is taken by the Pritikin Program, which emphasizes a complex carbohydrate, high fiber, and low fat diet. (See Chapter 5, *The Pritikin Program and Diabetes*.)

WHAT YOU NEED TO DO TO LOWER BLOOD CHOLESTEROL

The typical American diet is outrageously high in saturated fats. Dairy products, fried foods, cakes, hot dogs, hamburgers, and pizzas are examples of foods rich in cholesterol and saturated fats. Even a lean filet mignon with no visible white streaking has at least 30% fat content! It should come as no surprise that heart disease has reached epidemic proportions in this country. In pre–World War II Japan, the typical Japanese diet consisted of fruits and vegetables, rice, and fish. Heart disease at that time was extremely rare among the general population. With the postwar westernization of the Japanese diet, the incidence of heart disease has steadily risen. Hyperlipidemia, high lipid levels in the blood, is the key factor in the development of hardening of the arteries.

Now that you know about blood cholesterol, get set to lower it. All healthy Americans, regardless of their blood cholesterol level, should eat in a heart-healthy way. This is true beginning with children above age 5 on up to their parents, grandparents, and even great-grandparents. The whole family should also be physically active. And if you have a high blood cholesterol level—whether due to what you eat or to heredity—it is even more important to eat healthfully and to be physically active. Adopting these behaviors can help control high blood pressure as well as diabetes.

Here are some general rules to lower blood cholesterol:

Choose Foods Low in Saturated Fat

All foods that contain fat are made up of a mixture of saturated and unsaturated fats. Saturated fat raises your blood cholesterol level more than anything else that you eat. It is found in greatest amounts in foods from animals, such as fatty cuts of meat, poultry with the skin, whole-milk dairy products, lard, and in some vegetable oils like coconut, palm kernel, and palm oils. The best way to reduce your blood cholesterol level is to choose foods low in saturated fat. One way to do this is by choosing foods, such as fruit, vegetables, whole grain foods, breads, and cereals, naturally low in fat and high in starch and fiber.

Choose Foods Low in Total Fat

Since many foods high in total fat are also high in saturated fat, eating foods low in total fat will help you eat less saturated fat. When you do eat fat, you should substitute unsaturated fat for saturated fat. Unsaturated fat is usually liquid at room temperature and can be either monounsaturated or polyunsaturated. Examples of foods high in monounsaturated fat are olive and canola oils, those high in polyunsaturated fat, include safflower, sunflower, corn, and soybean oils. Any type of fat is a rich source of calories, so eating foods low in fat will also help you keep your weight under control.

Choose Foods High in Starch and Fiber

Foods high in starch and fiber are excellent substitutes for foods high in saturated fat. These foods—breads, cereals, pasta, grains, fruits, and vegetables—are low in saturated fat and cholesterol. They are also usually lower in calories than foods that are high in fat. Foods high in starch and fiber are also good sources of vitamins and minerals.

Diets low in saturated fat and cholesterol, and high in fruits, vegetables, and grain products—like oat and barley bran, and dry peas and beans—may help to lower blood cholesterol.

Choose Foods Low in Cholesterol

Dietary cholesterol also can raise your blood cholesterol level, although usually not as much as saturated fat. So, it is important to choose foods low in dietary cholesterol. Dietary cholesterol is found only in foods that come from animals. Many of these foods also are high in saturated fat. Foods from plant sources do not have cholesterol but can contain saturated fat.

Be More Physically Active

Being physically active helps your blood cholesterol levels: It can raise HDL and may lower LDL. Being more active also can help you lose weight, lower your blood pressure, improve the fitness of your heart and blood vessels, and reduce stress.

Lose Weight, if You are Overweight

People who are overweight tend to have higher blood cholesterol levels than people of desirable weight. And overweight people with an "apple" shape—bigger (pot) belly—tend to have a higher risk for heart disease than those with a "pear" shape—bigger hips and thighs.

Whatever your body shape, when you cut the fat in your diet, you cut down on the richest source of calories. An eating pattern high in starch and fiber instead of fat is a good way to lose weight. Starchy foods have little fat and are lower in calories than high-fat foods. If you are overweight, losing even a little weight can help to lower LDL cholesterol and raise HDL cholesterol. You don't need to reach your desirable weight to see a change in your blood cholesterol levels.

To Lower Your Blood Cholesterol, Remember to

- Choose foods low in saturated fat and cholesterol
- Be more physically active
- Lose weight, if you are overweight

Sources of Saturated Fat and Cholesterol

Animal fat	Hardened fat or oil
Bacon fat	Lamb fat
Beef fat	Lard
Butter	Meat fat
Chicken fat	Palm kernel oil
Cocoa butter	Pork fat
Coconut	Turkey fat
Coconut oil	Vegetable oil*
Cream	Vegetable shortening
Egg and egg yolk solids	Whole milk solids
Ham fat	

Read Food Labels

We have already mentioned that reading food labels will help you choose foods low in saturated fat, cholesterol, calories, and sodium. What will the labels tell you? Food labels have two important parts: the nutrition information and the ingredients list. Also, some labels have different claims like "low fat" or "light."

Read the nutrition information

Look for the amount of saturated fat, total fat, cholesterol, and calories in a serving of a product. Compare similar products to find the one with the smallest amounts. If you have high blood pressure, do the same for sodium.

*Could be coconut or palm oil

PRODUCT: CHECK FOR:

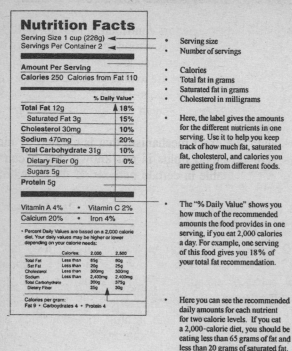

Nutrition Facts

Serving Size 1 cup (228g)
Servings Per Container 2

- Serving size
- Number of servings

Amount Per Serving
Calories 250 Calories from Fat 110

- Calories
- Total fat in grams
- Saturated fat in grams
- Cholesterol in milligrams

	% Daily Value*
Total Fat 12g	18%
Saturated Fat 3g	15%
Cholesterol 30mg	10%
Sodium 470mg	20%
Total Carbohydrate 31g	10%
Dietary Fiber 0g	0%
Sugars 5g	
Protein 5g	

- Here, the label gives the amounts for the different nutrients in one serving. Use it to help you keep track of how much fat, saturated fat, cholesterol, and calories you are getting from different foods.

Vitamin A 4%	•	Vitamin C 2%
Calcium 20%	•	Iron 4%

- The "% Daily Value" shows you how much of the recommended amounts the food provides in one serving, if you eat 2,000 calories a day. For example, one serving of this food gives you 18% of your total fat recommendation.

* Percent Daily Values are based on a 2,000 calorie diet. Your daily values may be higher or lower depending on your calorie needs:

	Calories:	2,000	2,500
Total Fat	Less than	65g	80g
Sat Fat	Less than	20g	25g
Cholesterol	Less than	300mg	300mg
Sodium	Less than	2,400mg	2,400mg
Total Carbohydrate		300g	375g
Dietary Fiber		25g	30g

Calories per gram:
Fat 9 • Carbohydrates 4 • Protein 4

- Here you can see the recommended daily amounts for each nutrient for two calorie levels. If you eat a 2,000-calorie diet, you should be eating less than 65 grams of fat and less than 20 grams of saturated fat. Your daily amounts may vary higher or lower depending on your calorie needs.

Look at the ingredients

All food labels list the product's ingredients in order by weight. The ingredient in the greatest amount is listed first. The ingredient in the least amount is listed last. So, to choose foods low in saturated fat or total fat, limit your use of products in which high-fat ingredients are listed first. If you are watching your sodium intake, do the same for salt.

DRUG THERAPY USED FOR DYSLIPIDEMIA

Regardless of the factors contributing to your high cholesterol, diet remains the keystone measure to correct this condition. If dietary measures are inadequate to achieve target goals, medications are available that can lower cholesterol and triglyceride levels. These medications require monitoring by your physician and are available only by prescription.

Niacin: The exact mechanism that is exerted by nicotinic acid on blood lipids is not known, but it can be extremely valuable in certain patients. If the patient can tolerate Niacin, this medication has the potential to accomplish lowering of LDL cholesterol and raising of HDL cholesterol, both of great benefit to diabetics who are prone to coronary heart disease. *However, because it may raise blood sugar, the use of niacin in diabetes is limited.*

Only about 40–50% of patients can remain on niacin because of rather severe side effects including marked reddening of the skin and itching, possible mild liver damage and gastrointestinal symptoms, and occasionally disturbances in cardiac rhythm.

Bile Acid Sequestrants (Questran, Colestid) are resins that bind with bile acids in the intestine and aid in their excretion in the feces. Cholesterol is the sole precursor of bile acids and inhibiting their absorption causes increased oxidation of cholesterol with subsequent decrease in blood LDL cholesterol. Side effects of these resins are constipation and some interference with absorption of certain medications and vitamins. They may also raise triglycerides.

Lorelco (Probucol) lowers total serum cholesterol, has little effect on triglycerides, and tends to *reduce* HDL cholesterol. It can be used in certain types of subgroups of dyslipidemia.

Lopid (Gemfibrozil) is the drug of choice for those with high blood triglycerides and although it has little effect on LDL cholesterol, it may increase HDL cholesterol. Its mechanism of action has not been definitely established.

HMG-CoA REDUCTASE INHIBITORS

The introduction of a new class of cholesterol-lowering drugs that work by interfering with the synthesis of cholesterol has revolutionized the treatment of dyslipidemia. The HMG-CoA reductase inhibitors, or "statins," have heralded a new era of treatment for hypercholesterolemia. Included in this category of drugs are Lovastatin (Mevacor), Simvastatin (Zocor), Fluvastatin (Lescol), Pravastatin (Pravachol), and Atorvastatin (Lipitor). Lipitor has been shown to have a beneficial effect in lowering the triglycerides as well as the LDL cholesterol. These pharmacological agents have proven to be safe, well tolerated, and very effective. Given in appropriate doses under medical supervision, this class of drugs has been shown in well documented studies to significantly lower the incidence of cardiovascular disease.

Pravastatin (Pravachol) therapy studies have shown prevention of acute coronary artery events (heart attacks and unstable angina) as early as six months to one year after instituting therapy. This short period of time for therapeutic effect may result from a physiological action independent of its cholesterol lowering properties. It has been theorized that this early protective benefit may be a result of stabilization of existing plaques as well as some, still as yet poorly understood biological alterations in the blood vessel wall.

As already noted, the stability of plaques and the condition of the inner lining of the blood vessel play major roles in acute coronary events. Plaque rupture explains the not infrequent acute coronary events in those with minor plaque formation (less than 30% occlusion of a coronary artery). This phenomenon also explains the sudden deaths in asymptomatic individuals who have an apparently normal electrocardiogram without clinical evidence of cardiovascular disease.

In short, stabilization of small plaques and improvement in the function of the blood vessel lining may explain this important early protective benefit of Pravachol as a phenomenon beyond its blood cholesterol lowering effect. Small asymptomatic plaque lesions are responsible for more than 80% of acute coronary events.

In November, 1994, the five-year Scandinavian Simvastin Survival Study (known as the 4 S Study) provided a controlled scientific look at more than 4,000 men who had either survived a heart attack or had angina pectoris (coronary insufficiency). The cholesterol level of the subjects averaged 260 mg/dl. The study had a double-blind, placebo-controlled format. The participants were divided into two groups. Half of them received Simvastatin and the other half were given placebo pills. The results clearly demonstrated the benefits of lowering blood cholesterol levels with medication. Those receiving the cholesterol-lowering drugs had a much lower incidence of coronary bypass surgery or balloon angiography, surgical treatments indicated for advanced coronary artery disease.

The overall mortality within the treated group was 30% less than in the control group. In other words, not only did far fewer patients require surgical intervention for advanced coronary disease, but the improved lipid level was accompanied by an overall improvement in health and decreased mortality.

In November 1995, Dr. James Shepherd of the University of Glasgow reported the results of the landmark Pravachol Primary Prevention Study (also known as the West of Scotland Coronary Prevention Study), in the prestigious New England Journal of Medicine. This double-blind, four-year study involved more than 6,500 Scottish men, aged 45–64, with cholesterol levels of 250–300 mg/dl with no known heart disease who were treated with pravastatin.

The results far exceeded the anticipated benefits of even the most optimistic proponents of drug intervention. The treated group had 33% fewer heart attacks, 20% fewer deaths from all causes, and 20% fewer bypass surgical procedures. The importance of treating a large segment of the population that has no known heart disease, but does have elevated cholesterol levels, was clearly demonstrated by the West of Scotland Study.

The study showed that drug intervention should be resorted to earlier than previously believed. If diet and exercise cannot achieve satisfactory reduction in abnormal lipid levels, drug therapy is definitely indicated. Those with additional risk factors are particularly vulnerable. These are the asymptomatic individuals with high lipid levels and silent underlying cardiovascular disease who may die without warning symptoms.

Cardiologist Dr. Eugene Braunwald, of Harvard and Boston's Brigham and Women's Hospital, is quite emphatic in his recommendations for the use of these drugs. "We're talking about a therapeutic revolution," Dr. Braunwald told a recent gathering of the American Heart Association in Orlando, Florida.

Patients on the "statins" must be monitored by their physician for adverse side effects such as elevated liver enzymes. In general, however, this class of drugs is well tolerated. The side effects are usually mild and reversible.

Blood tests to monitor liver function should be done periodically. Muscle inflammation, called myopathy, has been seen in less than one half of one percent of those on these medications.

The incidence of myopathy is increased when these drugs are taken along with Gemfibrozil or nicotinic acid at lipid-lowering doses (greater than one gram per day). The possible benefits of combined therapy with Gemfibrozil and a statin are not considered to be sufficient to outweigh the risk for developing myopathy. Patients with renal insufficiency, particularly the type associated with diabetes, are also at increased risk.

If you take a statin, you must familiarize yourself with the symptoms associated with myopathy: muscle aches or pains, and muscle tenderness or weakness, particularly if accompanied by malaise and fever. CPK is one of the blood enzyme tests performed periodically to monitor the statins. If the CPK level is elevated, or myopathy is suspected, the statin therapy must be discontinued.

With the loss of the protective effect of estrogens after menopause, the incidence of cardiovascular disease in postmenopausal women gradually rises until it approximates that of their male counterparts. Estrogen replacement therapy is of value in reducing coronary artery disease in women in this age group, if there are no medical contraindications to its use as determined by your physician.

ALCOHOL AND HEART DISEASE—THE FRENCH PARADOX

As long ago as 1819, Samuel Black, an Irish physician, noted that coronary artery disease was a not uncommon postmortem finding in his country, relatively rare in

France and the Mediterranean countries. He ascribed the discrepancy to some unknown differences in lifestyle or diet.

Despite the fact that the French eat three times as much saturated fat as their American counterparts, the incidence of coronary artery disease is only one-third of that in the United States. In 1991 this was the subject of a report on the CBS television show *60 Minutes*. The phenomenon became known popularly as the "French Paradox."

There are significant dietary differences between the eating habits in the two countries. The French drink less milk than Americans and eat more fresh vegetables, fruit, garlic, and cheese. They also consume considerably more wine.

Many epidemiologic studies have demonstrated that alcohol exerts some sort of protective effect against heart disease. The equivalent of two drinks per day has been shown to cause a significant decrease in heart disease. Higher doses of alcohol, however, are associated with an increased incidence of heart attacks and strokes. The protective effect of alcohol is to some degree associated with the ability of alcohol to raise the HDL cholesterol and prevent platelet agglutination. Red wine seems to have a particularly beneficial effect. The unique protective quality of red wine is believed to reside in its high content of flavinoids—powerful antioxidants—which are not present in white wine (except champagne) and are absent from beer with the exception of dark beers. Grape juice has about one half the amount of flavinoids as red wine.

Diabetics should get their flavinoids from sources other than wine. Onions and garlic are extremely high in antioxidant flavinoids that are heat stable and unaffected by cooking. Flavinoids are also found in tea (especially green tea) and all vegetables and fruits, particularly berries.

17

Long-Term Complications of Diabetes

- Neuropathy
- Cardiovascular Disease
- Retinopathy
- Nephropathy

Diabetes can affect many parts of the body. Over time it can damage a person's kidneys, eyes, nervous system, blood vessels, and heart. These long-term complications can result in kidney failure, vision loss, nerve damage, heart attacks, and strokes.

DIABETIC NEUROPATHY

What Is Diabetic Neuropathy?

Diabetic neuropathy is a nerve disorder caused by diabetes. Symptoms of neuropathy include numbness and sometimes pain in the hands, feet, or legs. Nerve damage caused by diabetes can also lead to problems with internal organs, such as the digestive track, heart, and sexual organs, causing indigestion, diarrhea or constipation, dizziness, bladder infections, and impotence. In some cases, neuropathy can flare up suddenly, causing weakness and weight loss. Depression may follow. While some treatments are available, a great deal of research is still needed to understand how diabetes affects the nerves and to find more effective treatments for this complication.

What Causes Diabetic Neuropathy?

Scientists do not know what causes diabetic neuropathy, but several factors are likely to contribute to the disorder. High blood glucose causes chemical changes in nerves. These changes impair the nerves' ability to transmit signals. High blood glucose also damages blood vessels that carry oxygen and nutrients to the nerves. In addition, inherited factors probably unrelated to diabetes may make some people more susceptible to nerve disease than others.

How high blood glucose leads to nerve damage is a subject of intense research. The precise mechanism is not known. Researchers have discovered that high glucose levels affect many metabolic pathways in the nerves, leading to an accumulation of a sugar called sorbitol and depletion of a substance called myoinositol. However, studies in humans have not shown convincingly that these changes are the mechanism that causes nerve damage.

How Common Is Diabetic Neuropathy?

People with diabetes can develop nerve problems at any time. Significant clinical neuropathy can develop within the first ten years after diagnosis of diabetes and the risk of developing neuropathy increases the longer a person has diabetes.

Diabetic neuropathy appears to be more common in smokers, people over forty years of age, and those who have had problems controlling their blood glucose levels.

More recently, researchers have focused on the effects of excessive glucose metabolism on the amount of nitrous oxide in nerves. Nitrous oxide dilates blood vessels. In a person with diabetes, low levels of nitrous oxide may lead to constriction of blood vessels supplying the nerve, contributing to nerve damage. Another promising area of research centers on the effect of glucose attaching to proteins when blood sugar is elevated, altering the structure and function of the proteins and affecting vascular function.

Scientists are studying how these changes occur, how they are connected, how they cause nerve damage, and how to prevent and treat damage.

What Are the Symptoms of Diabetic Neuropathy?

The symptoms of diabetic neuropathy vary. Numbness and tingling in feet are often the first signs. Some people notice no symptoms, while others are severely disabled. Neuropathy may cause both pain and insensitivity to pain in the same person. Often, symptoms are slight at first, and since most nerve damage occurs over a period of years, mild cases may go unnoticed for a long time. In some people, mainly those afflicted by focal neuropathy, the onset of pain may be sudden and severe.

What Are the Major Types of Neuropathy?

The symptoms of neuropathy also depend on which nerves and what part of the body is affected. Neuropathy may be diffuse, affecting many parts of the body, or focal, affecting a single, specific nerve and part of the body.

Diffuse Neuropathy

The two categories of diffuse neuropathy are peripheral neuropathy, affecting the feet and hands, and autonomic neuropathy, affecting the internal organs.

Peripheral Neuropathy

The most common type of peripheral neuropathy damages the nerves of the limbs, especially the feet. Nerves on both sides of the body are affected. Common symptoms of this kind of neuropathy are:

- Numbness or insensitivity to pain or temperature
- Tingling, burning, or prickling
- Extreme sensitivity to touch, even light touch
- Loss of balance and coordination

These symptoms are often worse at night. The damage to nerves often results in loss of reflexes and muscle weakness. The foot often becomes wider and shorter, the gait changes, and foot ulcers appear as pressure is put on parts of the foot that are less protected. Because of the loss of sensation, injuries may go unnoticed and often become infected. If ulcers or foot injuries are not treated in time, the infection may involve the bone and require amputation. However, problems caused by minor injuries can usually be controlled if they are caught in time. Avoiding foot injury by wearing well-fitted shoes and examining the feet daily can help prevent amputations.

Autonomic Neuropathy (also called visceral neuropathy)

Autonomic neuropathy is another form of diffuse neuropathy. It affects the nerves that serve the heart and internal organs and produces changes in many processes and systems.

Urination and sexual response: Autonomic neuropathy most often affects the organs that control urination and sexual function. Nerve damage can prevent the bladder from emptying completely, so bacteria grow more easily in the urinary tract (bladder and kidneys). When the nerves of the bladder are damaged, a person may have difficulty knowing when the bladder is full or controlling it, resulting in urinary incontinence.

The nerve damage and circulatory problems of diabetes can also lead to a gradual loss of sexual response in both men and women, although sex drive is unchanged. A man may be unable to have erections or may reach sexual climax without ejaculating normally.

Digestion

Autonomic neuropathy can affect digestion. Nerve damage can cause the stomach to empty too slowly, a disorder called gastric stasis. When the condition is severe (gastroparesis), a person can have persistent nausea and vomiting, bloating, and loss of appetite. Blood glucose levels tend to fluctuate greatly with this condition.

If nerves in the esophagus are involved, swallowing may be difficult. Nerve damage to the bowels can cause constipation or frequent diarrhea, especially at night. Problems with the digestive system often lead to weight loss.

Autonomic neuropathy can affect the cardiovascular system, which controls the circulation of blood throughout the body. Damage to this system interferes with the nerve impulses from various parts of the body that signal the need for blood and regulate blood pressure and heart rate. As a result, blood pressure may drop sharply after sitting and standing, causing a person to feel dizzy or light-headed, or even to faint (orthostatic hypotension).

Neuropathy that affects the cardiovascular system may also affect the perception of pain from heart disease. People may not experience angina as a warning sign of heart disease or may suffer painless heart attacks. It may also raise the risk of a heart attack during general anesthesia.

Autonomic neuropathy can hinder the body's normal response to low blood sugar or hypoglycemia, which makes it difficult to recognize and treat an insulin reaction.

Autonomic neuropathy can affect the nerves that control sweating. Sometimes, nerve damage interferes with the activity of the sweat glands, making it difficult for the body to regulate its temperature. Other times, the result can be profuse sweating at night or while eating (gustatory sweating).

Focal Neuropathy (including multiplex neuropathy)

Occasionally, diabetic neuropathy appears suddenly and affects specific nerves, most often in the torso, leg, or head. Focal neuropathy may cause:

- Pain in the front of a thigh
- Severe pain in the lower back or pelvis
- Pain in the chest, stomach, or flank
- Chest or abdominal pain sometimes mistaken for angina, heart attack, or appendicitis
- Aching behind an eye
- Inability to focus the eye
- Double vision
- Paralysis on one side of the face (Bell's palsy)
- Problems with hearing

This kind of neuropathy is unpredictable and occurs most often in older people who have mild diabetes. Although focal neuropathy can be painful, it tends to improve by itself after a period of weeks or months without causing long-term damage.

People with diabetes are also prone to developing compression neuropathies. The most common form of compression neuropathy is carpal tunnel syndrome. Asymptomatic carpal tunnel syndrome occurs in 20–30% of people with diabetes, and symptomatic carpal tunnel syndrome occurs in 6–11%. Numbness and tingling of the hand are the most common symptoms. Muscle weakness may also develop.

How Do Doctors Diagnose Diabetic Neuropathy?

A doctor diagnoses neuropathy based on symptoms and a physical exam. During the exam, the doctor may check muscle strength, reflexes, and sensitivity to position, vibration, temperature, and light touch. Sometimes special tests are also used to help determine the cause of symptoms and to suggest treatment.

A simple *screening test* to check point sensation in the feet can be done in the doctor's office. The test uses a nylon filament mounted on a small wand. The filament delivers a standardized 10-gram force when touched to areas of the foot. Patients who cannot sense pressure from the filament have lost protective sensation and are at risk for developing neuropathic foot ulcers.

Nerve conduction studies check the flow of electrical current through a nerve. With this test, an image of the nerve impulse is projected on a screen as it transmits an electrical signal. Impulses that seem slower or weaker than usual indicate possible damage to the nerve. This test allows the doctor to assess the condition of all the nerves in the arms and legs.

Electromyography (*EMG*) is used to see how well muscles respond to electrical impulses transmitted by nearby nerves. The electrical activity of the muscle is displayed on a screen. A response that is slower or weaker than usual suggests damage to the nerve or muscle. This test is often done at the same time as nerve conduction studies.

Ultrasound employs sound waves. The sound waves are too high to hear, but they produce an image showing how well the bladder and other parts of the urinary tract are functioning.

Nerve biopsy involves removing a sample of nerve tissue for examination. This test is most often used in research settings.

If your doctor suspects autonomic neuropathy, you may also be referred to a physician who specializes in digestive disorders (gastroenterologist) for additional tests.

How Is Diabetic Neuropathy Usually Treated?

Treatment aims to relieve discomfort and prevent further tissue damage. The first step is to bring blood sugar under control by diet and oral drugs or insulin injections, if needed, and by careful monitoring of blood sugar levels. Although symptoms can sometimes worsen at first as blood sugar is brought under control, maintaining lower blood sugar levels helps reverse the pain or loss of sensation that neuropathy can cause. Good control of blood sugar may also help prevent or delay the onset of further problems.

Another important part of treatment involves special care of the feet, which are prone to problems. (See Chapter 20, *Care of the Feet*.)

A number of medications and other approaches are used to relieve the symptoms of diabetic neuropathy.

Relief of Pain

For relief of pain, burning, tingling, or numbness, the doctor may suggest an analgesic such as aspirin or acetaminophen or antiinflammatory drugs containing ibuprofen. Nonsteroidal antiinflammatory drugs should be used with caution in people with renal disease. Antidepressant medications such as amitriptyline (sometimes used with fluphenazine) or nerve medications such as carbamazepine or phenytoin sodium may be helpful. Codeine is sometimes prescribed for short-term use to relieve severe pain. In addition, a topical cream, capsaicin, is now available to help relieve the pain of neuropathy.

Other treatments include hypnosis, relaxation training, biofeedback, and acupuncture. Some people find that walking regularly or using elastic stockings helps relieve leg pain. Warm (not hot) baths, massage, or an analgesic ointment may also help. After age forty, *never* massage your legs. Many adults have asymptomatic blood clots in their deep veins that will never cause a problem unless they are dislodged by vigorous manipulation such as massage therapy.

Gastrointestinal Problems

Indigestion, belching, nausea, or vomiting are symptoms of gastroparesis. For patients with mild symptoms of slow stomach emptying, doctors suggest eating small, frequent meals and avoiding fats. Eating less fiber may also relieve symptoms. For patients with severe gastroparesis, the doctor may prescribe metoclopramide, which speeds digestion and helps relieve nausea. Other drugs that help regulate digestion or reduce stomach acid secretion may also be used. In each case, the potential benefits of these drugs need to be weighed against their side effects.

To avoid diarrhea or other bowel problems, antibiotics or clonidine HC1, a drug used to treat high blood pressure, are sometimes prescribed. The antibiotic tetracycline may be prescribed. A wheat-free diet may also bring relief since the gluten in flour sometimes causes diarrhea.

Neurological problems affecting the urinary tract can result in infections or incontinence. The doctor may prescribe an antibiotic to clear up an infection and suggest drinking more fluids to prevent further infections. If incontinence is a problem, patients may be advised to urinate at regular times (every three hours, for example) since they may not be able to tell when the bladder is full.

Dizziness, Weakness

Sitting or standing slowly may help prevent lightheadedness, dizziness, or fainting, which are symptoms that may be associated with some forms of autonomic neuropathy. Raising the head of the bed and wearing elastic stockings may also help.

Muscle weakness or loss of coordination caused by diabetic neuropathy can often be helped by physical therapy.

Urinary and Sexual Problems

Nerve and circulatory problems of diabetes can disrupt normal male sexual function, resulting in impotence. After ruling out a hormonal cause of impotence, the doctor can provide information about methods available to treat impotence caused by neuropathy. Short-term solutions involve using a mechanical vacuum device or injecting a drug called a vasodilator into the penis before sex. A vasodilatory medication in suppository form that works efficiently is now available. (See Chapter 21, *Diabetes and Impotence.*) Surgical procedures, in which an inflatable or semirigid device is implanted in the penis, offers a more permanent solution. For some people, counseling may help relieve the stress caused by neuropathy and thereby help restore sexual function.

In women who feel their sexual life is not satisfactory, the role of diabetic neuropathy is less clear. Illness, vaginal or urinary tract infections, and anxiety about pregnancy complicated by diabetes can interfere with a woman's ability to enjoy intimacy. Infections can be reduced by good blood glucose control. Counseling may also help a woman identify and cope with sexual concerns.

Why Is Good Foot Care Important for People With Diabetic Neuropathy?

People with diabetes need to take special care of their feet. Neuropathy and blood vessel disease both increase the risk of foot ulcers. The nerves to the feet are the longest in the body, and are most often affected by neuropathy. Because of the loss of sensation caused by neuropathy, sores or injuries to the feet may not be noticed and may become ulcerated.

At least 15% of all people with diabetes eventually have a foot ulcer, and 6 out of every 1,000 people with diabetes have an amputation. However, doctors estimate that nearly three-quarters of all amputations caused by neuropathy and poor circulation could be prevented with careful foot care. Read the rules for foot care spelled out in Chapter 20, *Care of the Feet.*

Are There Any Experimental Treatments for Diabetic Neuropathy?

Several new drugs under study may eventually prevent or reverse diabetic neuropathy. However, extensive testing is required by the U.S. Food and Drug Administration to establish the safety and efficacy of drugs before they are approved for widespread use.

Researchers are exploring treatment with a compound called myoinositol. Early findings have shown that nerves in diabetic animals and humans have less than normal amounts of this substance. Myoinositol supplements increase the levels of this substance in tissues of diabetic animals, but research is still needed to show any concrete lasting benefits from this treatment.

Another area of research concerns the drug aminoguanidine. In animals, this drug blocks cross-linking of proteins that occurs more quickly than normal in tissues exposed to high levels of glucose. Early clinical tests are under way to determine the effects of aminoguanidine in humans.

One approach that appeared promising involved the use of aldose reductase inhibitors (ARIs). ARIs are a class of drugs that block the formation of the sugar alcohol sorbitol, which is thought to damage nerves. Scientists hoped these drugs would prevent and might even repair nerve damage. But so far, clinical trials have shown that these drugs have major side effects and, consequently, are not available for clinical use.

Diabetic Neuropathy Can Affect Virtually Every Part of the Body

Diffuse (Peripheral) Neuropathy
- Legs
- Feet
- Arms
- Hands

Diffuse (Autonomic) Neuropathy
- Heart
- Digestive system
- Sexual organs
- Urinary tract
- Sweat glands

Focal Neuropathy
- Eyes
- Facial muscles
- Hearing
- Pelvis and lower back
- Thighs
- Abdomen

CARDIOVASCULAR DISEASE

Arteriosclerotic heart disease is the number one killer in the United States. As many as one-third to one-half of patients with heart attacks demonstrate abnormal glucose metabolism or have a definitive diagnosis of diabetes. The Framingham Heart Disease Study has shown that diabetes, along with other risk factors such as high blood pressure and smoking, is a major factor in the increased incidence of heart and cardiovascular disease.

The inner lining (the basement membrane) of capillaries has been the object of study for many years by researchers attempting to determine the link between diabetes and blood vessel disease. It has been found that more than 90% of adult diabetics have an abnormal capillary basement membrane. In addition, researchers found that non-diabetic close relatives of diabetics have a 50% chance of having thickened capillary membranes as well. These findings confirm the hypothesis that genetic as well as metabolic factors are the underlying cause of the cardiovascular complications found in diabetes.

The high incidence of dyslipidemia in diabetics is one of the major causes of premature atherosclerosis and cardiovascular disease. The older one becomes, the more cholesterol is deposited in the walls of blood vessels and the more severe the atherosclerotic process. Accordingly, those above forty have a greater risk of developing heart attacks, strokes, or any of the other sequelae and complications of atherosclerosis. (See Chapter 16, *Diabetes, Lipids, and Atherosclerosis.*)

While diabetics have a higher risk of coronary, cerebral, and peripheral vascular disease, the risk can be sharply decreased by rigid control of blood sugar, adherence to a low-fat, low-cholesterol diet, regular exercise, maintaining good hygiene, and avoiding stress on a daily basis.

DIABETIC RETINOPATHY

Blindness is one of the most feared complications of long-standing diabetes. It is true that diabetes mellitus is the leading cause of blindness in the United States. The incidence of blindness from diabetic retinopathy is 0.2%

per year in all diabetics, but this fact may be somewhat misleading. "Legal" blindness is defined as vision 20/200 or less and does not necessarily mean total blindness. A person may be legally blind and still be able to perform most of his daily chores with the exception of driving and tasks that obviously require more acute vision. In fact, not more than 5% of the diabetic population is completely blind. This low figure is a result of new and modern scientific treatments available for diabetic eye problems.

The eye is actually a small sphere filled with a clear gel called the vitreous. The retina is a delicate membrane of nerve tissue that lines the inside of the eye chamber. It acts like a photographic film that receives visual stimuli and transmits the "picture" to the brain for interpretation. This visual impulse passes along the optic nerve and goes directly to the visual center located in the back of the brain. Indeed, the optic nerve itself is a direct extension of the brain.

Your doctor can visualize the inside of the eye and the optic nerve with an instrument called an ophthalmoscope. The tiny blood vessels that provide nourishment to the eye can be seen radiating out from this optic disc. With long-standing diabetes, these retinal vessels can weaken and subsequently develop tiny "blow outs" called microaneurysms that can leak plasma out of the confines of the tiny capillary. In some, this is followed by the formation of new blood vessels associated with scar formation of the damaged tissues, resulting in visual loss.

The above sequence of events is given the generic name, *diabetic retinopathy*. Retinopathy can be divided into two major categories: *nonproliferative* or background retinopathy and *proliferative* retinopathy. The former includes venous abnormalities, microaneurysms, retinal bleeding, and accumulations of lipid or protein containing fluid called exudates. The abnormality in non-proliferative retinopathy can be seen with a procedure known as fluorescein angiography and often can be reversed with excellent glucose control. Edema of the retina is due to abnormal capillary permeability and poor blood supply (ischemia). "Macular" edema is a serious complication and must be treated early by photocoagulation. This treatment will be discussed later.

The hallmark of *proliferative* retinopathy is new blood vessel formation (neovascularization). These tiny vascular loops grow on the surface of the retina or extend into the vitreous. Traction may develop between the vitreous and the neovascular elements leading to another serious complication, retinal detachment. A table showing the types of diabetic retinopathy follows:

A. Background retinopathy or nonproliferative retinopathy
1. Microaneurysms with or without tiny hemorrhages
2. Exudates (hard)
3. Venous and arteriolar abnormalities
4. Retinal edema

B. Preproliferative retinopathy
1. Soft exudates or "cotton wool" spots
2. Intra-retinal vascular abnormalities
3. Areas of "nonperfusion"
4. Macular edema

C. Proliferative Retinopathy
1. New vessels on the optic disc
2. New vessels in other areas
3. Growth of fibrous tissue
4. Contraction of fibrous tissue with retinal hemorrhage or retinal detachment

Don't let these terms scare you. Actually, non-proliferative or background retinopathy usually does not interfere with vision except when there is an accumulation of fluid in the macular area, and this complication is now treated early and quite successfully. Remember, most of these conditions can be adequately treated and only 5% of diabetics go on to complete loss of vision.

Type I diabetics usually develop mild reversible changes such as some leakage of retinal vessels within a few years of onset of abnormally high glucose levels. In approximately ten years, they will usually have microaneurysms and some exudate on the retina that can be visualized with the ophthalmoscope by the attending physician. With poor control of blood sugars, hemorrhages, fibrous tissue, and some dimming of vision may occur because of changes in the retina.

The retinal changes in Type II diabetes have an unpredictable course and may go unnoticed for years. This is why careful examination of the eyes on each medical visit is important to document any progressive changes in order to note the development of tiny hemorrhages or exudate on the retina.

Diabetics may experience temporary blurring of vision and changes in refraction most likely due to osmotic changes in the shape of the lens as a result of fluctuations in blood sugars. While uncomfortable, new refractions and glasses for the eyes should not be obtained until a steady period of glucose control occurs. It may take six to eight weeks before the changes in visual acuity become stabilized.

Remember, every visual defect in the diabetic is not necessarily a consequence of retinopathy. Eye disorders that occur in the general population, such as glaucoma, cataracts, and conjunctivitis, occur with increased frequency in diabetes. Glaucoma (increased pressure in the interior of the eye) is particularly common in older diabetic patients.

Treatment of Diabetic Retinopathy

Studies have shown that rigid control of blood sugars can ameliorate the optic nerve and vascular changes seen in diabetes. Animal research seems to indicate that good control of glucose can slow or even stop the progression of retinopathy. "Tight" control of diabetes, as with all the acute and chronic complications of this disease, is imperative to slow down progression.

Photocoagulation is a method of focusing a light beam on the retina to produce a burn or coagulation in a precisely defined area. This allows the ophthalmologist to destroy microaneurysms, leaky vessels, neovascular areas, and areas of edema. This prevents further deterioration. It has been shown by trials carried out by the Diabetic Retinopathy Study Research Group that photocoagulation decreases the incidence of retinal detachment, hemorrhage, and loss of vision. While the Argon Laser has proved to be a valuable tool for photocoagulation, newer and better instruments are presently in use in many centers specializing in retinal diseases. A procedure called vitrectomy can be performed when necessary in severe cases to remove hemorrhagic and fibrous tissue blocking vision. This procedure involves introducing a hollow needle, with a cutting device attached, into the vitreous and removing the material affecting vision. The vitreous gel is replaced with a saline solution. This operation has proven very helpful in patients who have an accumulation of material interfering with vision. Only highly trained ophthalmologists are qualified to perform this delicate operation.

The Diabetes Control and Complications Trial (DCCT)

showed that with "intensive control" patients had a 76% reduction in the risk of retinopathy. This finding stands as a motivating factor to all diabetic patients who want to avoid future visual problems. Careful examination and evaluation of your eyes by your diabetologist and ophthalmologist can initiate early treatment if necessary and prevent many of the major visual complications of diabetes.

Note: Opticians are called "doctor," but they do not have the medical training to evaluate and treat medical problems of the eyes. Even family practitioners and diabetologists are limited in their ability to visualize the retina. Only ophthalmalogists have the equipment and expertise to visualize more than 95% of the retina on fundoscopic exam and render treatment early enough to successfully prevent or reverse eye damage. Diabetics should be monitored on a regular basis by their ophthalmologist.

DIABETIC NEPHROPATHY

The kidneys filter the waste products from the blood while preserving the important elements the body requires for future use. When protein is metabolized, nitrogenous waste products are produced that are eliminated by the kidneys. Nephropathy refers to changes in the kidneys due to infection, hardening of the small arteries that nourish the kidneys, and damage to the filtering systems within the kidney tissue. With progressive diabetic damage, protein, which is usually conserved by the kidney, begins to appear in tiny amounts in the urine. The excretion of the microscopic protein (albumin) is an important measurement that can serve as an early indicator in detecting beginning pathologic changes in the kidney. It can also be used as a guide to monitor the rate of progression of renal disease. Persistent microalbumin levels of 20–200 micrograms or more over a six-month period indicate a diagnosis of early diabetic nephropathy. The thickening of the basement membrane, described earlier as a part of vascular disease, also takes place in the renal vessels and accounts for much of the gradual deterioration of kidney function, leading to end-stage renal disease. Experimental evidence strongly suggests that persistently elevated blood sugars play a major role in causing diabetic nephropathy. Islet cell transplant experiments done in rodents have resulted in marked reduction in the pathologic changes seen in diabetic nephropathy. The key to treating nephropathy is to control the blood pressure, to strictly manage blood sugars, and to decrease the workload of the kidneys by placing the patient on a low-protein diet along with "tight" management of blood glucose.

When end-stage nephropathy reaches the point of threatening the way of life and even possibly proving fatal to the diabetic patient, renal dialysis or kidney transplant can compensate for, or take the place of, the patient's own failing kidneys.

Thus, there are treatment modalities available now that will extend longevity to diabetics with advanced nephropathy and allow a return to a near-normal existence.

HYPERTENSION AND DIABETES

Hypertension occurs with greater frequency in both Type I and Type II diabetics than in the population at large. Uncontrolled diabetes not only contributes to the accelerated atherosclerotic process that often accompanies diabetes, but also plays a prominent role in the frequently associated high blood pressure. However, atherosclerosis alone does not explain the high rate of hypertension found in diabetics except in those instances when there is moderate to severe involvement of the blood supply to the kidneys caused by the atheromatous changes.

It has been theorized that the hypertension may, in some way, be related to the "insulin resistance" that is found not only in diabetics but also in the obese. In fact, maturity-onset diabetes is often accompanied by "insulin resistance," obesity, and hypertension. As discussed previously, insulin resistance is related to decreased receptors for insulin at the cellular level, decreased binding of insulin to the cell membrane, and difficulty transporting glucose across the cell membrane into the cell to provide energy.

Another finding related to high blood pressure in the diabetic is increased sodium retention by the kidney, leading to increased blood volume and eventually damage to the kidney's filtering function.

Tight glucose control has been shown to reduce microalbuminuria or proteinuria. The test for microalbumin is now an essential part of the examination of all diabetic patients. A family history of hypertension should make the physician and patient more aware of potential nephropathy-associated high blood pressure.

Control of blood pressure has a definite ameliorating effect on kidney function. A wide array of medications are available that effectively lower blood pressure in almost all cases.

There are several major classes of antihypertensive drugs available. Many physicians feel that aldosterone-converting enzyme inhibitors (ACE inhibitors) have a favorable effect in diabetics by reducing the "hyperfiltration" in the kidneys that accompanies the diabetic state. However, there are some important contraindications to this form of therapy. Diuretics reduce the increased blood volume and blood pressure but have other possible adverse side effects. Beta-blockers, calcium channel blockers, and a markedly decreased salt intake are all available to patients who have been diagnosed with hypertension. The physician must take into account factors such as race, age, and other cardiovascular and renal diseases before prescribing a specific medicine for the diabetic with high blood pressure. The diabetes must be kept under control by utilizing glucose monitoring as well as laboratory glycohemoglobin determinations approximately every eight weeks. Examination of the retina and palpation of the pulse in the lower legs is routine in hypertensive patients. Diet and weight control play important roles in the management of the hypertensive diabetic patient. Obesity makes control of high blood pressure more difficult. Prohibition of smoking is of extreme importance as well as enforcing a low-salt, low-saturated fat diet. If blood lipids are high, additional medications to lower total cholesterol and low-density cholesterol (LDL) and raise high-density cholesterol (HDL) are in order.

In summary, the problems of hypertension and concomitant cardiovascular problems are more prevalent in the diabetic than in the general population. The patient and the doctor must be willing to work together to control the blood sugar, keep the blood pressure within normal range, treat hyperlipidemia if present, and keep weight within normal limits. While these endeavors may require constant vigil, the long-term results will make the effort worthwhile.

18

Travel and the Diabetic

• Planning a Trip
• Equipment to Take When Traveling
• Necessary Precautions

Diabetes should not interfere with travel. By taking simple precautions, you can enjoy the mountains, museums, camping, athletic events, cruises, and participate with others on exciting tours and visits to foreign lands and meet people of many cultures.

All travelers have the opportunity and pleasure of planning their vacation as well as preparing for glitches or emergencies that may arise. Diabetic patients have an even greater obligation to plan ahead, check the areas they will be visiting, obtain knowledge in advance of the medical facilities available, and make certain to bring adequate supplies of medications, syringes, insulin, and any other items their doctor recommends for the trip. When asked, physicians usually will provide their patients with a medical report of their history, a list of medications, and significant information for other medical personnel, if the need for treatment should arise. The report will also help to avoid problems with police or custom officials who may wish to know why there are drugs and/or syringes in your luggage. Your doctor can prescribe medications in advance for treatment of minor common ailments such as diarrhea, mild gastrointestinal symptoms, or colds. All travelers arriving in new surroundings and cultures should avoid eating unpeeled fruits, leafy vegetables, under-cooked meats, cheeses, or cream sauces. It is wise to avoid local drinking water unless you are certain it is safe. Montezuma's revenge has been experienced by many U.S. visitors to Mexico. It is interesting to note that Mexican visitors to the U.S. also often experience bouts of diarrhea from local water supplies that meet strict public health standards. This occurs because each country has its own unique strains of bacteria that cause problems when you are not accustomed to them.

The names and addresses of competent medical providers can be obtained, before starting your trip. The International Association for Assistance to Medical Travelers is a nonprofit organization located at 417 Center Street, Lewiston, NY 14092. They publish a directory that lists addresses and phone numbers of English-speaking physicians throughout the world, whose qualifications and standards are deemed satisfactory. The Public Health Service in most communities can also give free advice regarding the need for required immunization procedures and information regarding endemic diseases in various parts of the world. Make certain you receive any necessary immunizations well in advance of your departure. This will allow adequate time to deal with any side effects, including interference with your diabetes control. If you are prone to motion sickness be sure to take along preventative medications. The American Diabetes Association offers information regarding physicians and medical facilities in the areas you intend to visit. In an urgent situation, American embassies often are of great help in obtaining prompt and qualified medical attention.

Check with your insurance carrier before your trip to ascertain coverage should the need for emergency medical or surgical care arise.

If you are unfamiliar with the local language, carry a phrase book or pocket computer-translator. Most countries measure blood sugar levels in milligrams per deciliter (mg/dl) as is done in the United States. However, in the United Kingdom and some other countries, the Systeme Internationale is used. Blood sugars are reported in millimols/liter (mM/1). To convert mg/dl to mM/1, divide by 18. Conversely, to change mM/1 to mg/dl, multiply by 18.

When buying your boat or plane ticket, always request a diabetic diet. If this service is not provided, you may order a regular diet and use your own knowledge and judgment in deciding which foods would have the least impact on your blood sugar levels.

Wearing a medic-alert medallion and identification bracelet is always desirable, but even more so when traveling in strange and exotic places. Medic-Alert, P.O. Box 1009, Turlock, CA 93581-1009, is a nonprofit organization that can help you to obtain materials to communicate vital medical information. It is prudent to take extra supplies of all items related to your diabetes when traveling. This includes your testing devices for blood sugar, extra batteries for glucose monitoring meters, lancets, test strips, alcohol, cotton, Band-Aids, syringes, vials of insulin, and soap for washing hands and cleansing the skin.

Be sure to take into account changes in time zones when traveling long distances. Discussion with your doctor or diabetic educator regarding changes in the timing and dosage of insulin is in order for trips that will cross several time zones. Upon arrival, you can adjust your meal and insulin schedule based on local time. Having your glucose test meter along will make it easier to regulate your blood sugar levels regardless of the changes in local time, climate, and diverse food availability.

Luggage can be misplaced or lost. It is vitally important

that your diabetic supplies, along with your wallet, passport, hotel and train reservations, and money are kept in a carry-on bag, not in checked luggage. Your carry-on bag should be secure and always under close observation. Crime exists all over the world. It is better to be safe than sorry. Divide your insulin and other diabetes supplies between two different bags. Then, if a bag is misplaced, you won't have lost all of your supplies. Your type, brand, species, and concentration of insulin(s) may not be available in other countries. Having to switch insulins in the middle of your trip could affect control. Be sure to bring along sufficient supplies to last the entire trip.

Whenever possible, keep insulin refrigerated between use. However, insulin that is not refrigerated remains stable for one month provided it is kept in a cool place (below 86 degrees F). Make sure it does not get too hot or too cold. Never leave your insulin in a parked car. Pack your insulin between layers of clothing in a bag you will be hand carrying. Store your insulin in a refrigerator as soon as possible after arriving. If refrigeration is not available, keeping your insulin in a wide-mouth insulated thermos can help. Fill the bottle with cold water or ice to cool it. Pour the cold water or ice out. Put the insulin vials inside the bottle and tighten the cap. *Insulin should never be frozen.* Allow insulin to warm to room temperature to avoid painful injections.

Outside the United States, U-100 syringes may not be available. Be sure to bring enough injection supplies with you. If you are going to visit a country where English is not spoken, carry an "I Have Diabetes" identification card in the local language and try to learn enough phrases to enable you to order meals, describe emergencies, and get medical care. Keep carbohydrate snacks available for those unforeseen delays in obtaining regular meals.

You will want to continue some form of exercise program while away from home. This may take the form of walking while sight-seeing and visiting museums and art galleries. Alternating your footwear with an extra pair of comfortable shoes will help to prevent sore feet and calluses.

Traveling companions and friends should know about your diabetes in order that they can be of assistance should the need arise. Be sure to take a glucagon kit with you and instruct one of your traveling companions in its use.

If you are traveling long distances by car, stop every few hours for short walks to aid circulation. Prolonged sitting, particularly for those over the age of forty, interferes with the circulation of the lower extremities and predisposes to phlebitis, a potentially dangerous condition.

Thousands of diabetic patients who have traveled the world over report that they have had exciting times and wonderful experiences without concerns as long as they planned ahead and took the few common sense precautionary steps described in this chapter.

19

Hygiene

- • **Dental Care**
- • **Skin Care**
- • **Foot Care**
- • **Eye Care**
- • **Urinary Tract Infections**

Uncontrolled elevated blood sugar levels increase the risk of infections, as well as interfering with wound healing. For this reason, it is important that you familiarize yourself with the simple precautions to be taken in the routine of daily life to prevent, whenever possible, future bothersome complications.

Hygiene is the art of the preservation of physical health. Diabetics must take special care of their skin, hair, eyes, teeth, and feet. Daily routines should be established to allow adequate time for meals, exercise, recreation, rest, and sleep. Emotional stresses such as worry and anxiety have the physiological effect of raising blood sugar, making control more difficult. The following sections outline the steps you must take for satisfactory personal care.

CARE OF THE SKIN

The skin, particularly that of the hands, may harbor bacteria that can cause infections. Bathe at least once daily with mild soap and water. Protect your skin by avoiding scratches or punctures by wearing gloves when you work at tasks that might injure your hands. Treat all injuries promptly. Wash cuts with warm, soapy water and apply a dry sterile dressing. Notify your doctor if cuts or scrapes show any signs of infection (redness, heat, swelling, tenderness, throbbing, or pus formation). If an infection does occur, use an antiseptic soap like Betadine that kills skin bacteria and may prevent the spread of infection.

The use of baby powder, particularly in areas where the skin rubs together, helps to prevent irritation. After a shower or swimming, drying the ear canals may help avert bacterial or fungal infection. Avoid sunburn by using sunscreen and common sense. Prevent frostbite by dressing wisely and avoiding excessive exposure during the cold weather. Select hypoallergenic deodorants and cosmetics. At the first sign of increased sensitivity, change to another brand. Women should not shave their legs with a safety razor; an electric razor is preferable. Chapping of hands can be prevented by thorough drying and the use of a bland cream. Fingernails should be kept the proper length. The cuticle may be gently pushed back with an orangewood stick, never with a pointed instrument.

CARE OF THE HAIR

The hair should be shampooed at least once or twice weekly with a hypoallergenic commercial preparation. Haircuts, shaves, and removal of hair should be done with scrupulously clean instruments.

CARE OF THE TEETH AND GUMS

Proper care of the teeth and gums is an excellent example of how simple daily prophylactic measures can prevent long-term problems.

Elevated blood sugar levels can affect all the tissues of the body, including the gums and teeth. There is a higher incidence of plaque and bacteria in the mouth and gums in uncontrolled diabetics. In addition, the proclivity of capillary blood vessels to narrow and deliver less oxygen and nourishment to the gum tissues leads to delay in healing of tiny cuts or bruises made by too vigorous brushing of the teeth or other trauma inflicted by such objects as hard candies, fish bones, or leathery and fibrous foods. Use only soft bristle toothbrushes. Hard bristles are prone to cause minor gum irritations, which can lead to periodontal disease.

While diabetes probably does not initiate periodontal or gum disease, it does delay the healing process and makes good dental care critical.

A dental abscess or severe periodontal disease can exacerbate the underlying diabetic condition by contributing to infection, interfering with proper eating, and causing stress, all tending to raise blood sugar levels.

Patients should be sure their dentist is aware of their diabetic status. The dentist or the dental hygienist can then give proper instructions regarding dental care: brushing, using floss, and massaging the gums periodically. The diabetic patient should make an appointment to visit his dentist at least every four to six months. When canker sores or painful, reddened gums occur, the dentist should be promptly notified.

Brush and floss every day after meals. Some dentists prefer the Water Pik to reduce the formation of plaque while others instruct the patient in the use of electrically operated toothbrushes. Circular or round movements of the brush at the gum line and over the tooth surface using toothpaste containing special ingredients will reduce plaque formation. It will also aid in keeping the teeth and gums and the bone structure underneath the gums healthy. Dentists recommend strict control of blood sugars before rendering any dental treatment—including even such minor procedures as dental cleaning or minor fillings. Before beginning intensive dental or gum treatment, antibiotics may be prescribed to prevent infection as well as the possibility of bacteremia—release of bacteria into the bloodstream as a result of dental manipulation.

Blood on the toothbrush or noted in expectorated saliva may be the first sign of gingivitis. A special type of gingivitis due to the herpes simplex virus can cause inflammation and bleeding that may be particularly severe in diabetes. Most of these infections are self-limited and require only symptomatic therapy, but antibiotics may be necessary to treat secondary infections.

Infections of the gums or roots of the teeth (endodontal infections) are usually associated with the rarer strains of anaerobic bacteria and are best treated by an endodontist.

REVIEW OF DENTAL CARE AND DIABETES

Although diabetics are not necessarily more prone to infection than non-diabetics, once an infection does develop, it tends to be more severe and last a longer period of time. Probably one of the most common types of chronic infection is inflammatory periodontal (gum) disease. It is also called pyorrhea, periodontitis, or gingivitis. Gingivitis is the beginning stage of gum disease in which the soft tissue surrounding the teeth becomes inflamed. If the inflammation extends to include the supporting bone surrounding the teeth, the condition is then called periodontitis.

Please keep in mind that it is not the frequency of cleaning the teeth, as much as how effectively you do the job, that is important. Proper cleaning techniques should be provided by your dentist or dental hygienist.

CARE OF THE EYES

The eye damage that diabetes may cause was discussed in Chapter 17, *Long-Term Complications of Diabetes*. Take the steps listed below to further reduce the risk and the danger of eye problems.

- Have a complete eye exam every year. Remember, eye damage has *no* symptoms in the early, most treatable stages.
- Visit an ophthalmologist, a medical doctor who specializes in eye care, at once if you have any of these symptoms of physical damage:
    blurred or double vision
    narrowed field of vision
    seeing dark spots
    feeling of pressure or pain in the eyes
    difficulty seeing in dim light
- Have your blood pressure checked often.
- Do not smoke.

URINARY TRACT INFECTIONS

Women with diabetes are especially prone to urinary tract infections. The lower urinary tract consists of the bladder, which collects the urine, and the urethra, the canal through which the urine is voided. The most common lower urinary tract infection occurs when bacteria gain entry to the bladder from the outside through the urethra, causing what is called cystitis. Common symptoms of cystitis are any or all of the following: urinary frequency, a constant desire to urinate even within a short time of having done so, straining at the end of urination, feelings that the bladder has not been completely emptied, burning with urination, and decreased strength of the urinary stream.

Anatomically, women are susceptible to bladder infections because the female urethra is a rather short channel that is located close to the vagina and rectum. The rectum, because of bowel movements, is a source of bacteria that can contaminate the urethra and enter the bladder. Once bacteria get into the vaginal area, entry into the bladder is easy, again because the urethra is an extremely short channel. Prompt and adequate treatment of urinary tract infections is essential to effect a complete cure and prevent recurrence.

There are a number of measures you can take to prevent urinary tract infections:

1. **Good Hygiene**—Always keep the area around the vagina and rectum clean and dry.
2. **Good Toilet Habits**—Improper wiping of the vaginal/rectal area after using the toilet can result in urinary tract infections. Always wipe from front to back, never the reverse, to avoid contamination of the vaginal-urethral area.
3. **Urinate Frequently**—Urinate regularly every three to four hours. This helps to prevent infection because it serves to flush out the bladder and urethra as well as avoiding overstretching of the bladder. When the bladder is full and forced to hold an unusual amount of fluid, minimal tissue damage to the wall of the bladder can result, making it more vulnerable to bacterial infection.

4. **Correct Wearing Apparel**—Bodysuits, pantyhose, or tight slacks should not be worn for long periods of time. They promote warm, moist, dark environments that are favorable sites for bacterial growth.

Sexual activity can play an important role in urinary tract infections. The roof of the vagina and the floor of the bladder is a very thin septum. Prolonged intercourse can contribute to tissue damage and predispose to bladder infections. This is particularly common in newlyweds and is well known to interns who refer to the condition as "honeymoon cystitis." During intercourse, bacteria in the vagina may be introduced into the urethra as a consequence of the motion associated with intercourse. Sexually active women can help to prevent infection by showering before intercourse, or at least washing the genital area thoroughly with soap and water. Always urinate after intercourse. This serves as an effective method to wash out any bacteria that may have gained entry into the urethra.

20

Care of the Feet

- How to Avoid Ulcers and Infections
- Importance of Early Diagnosis and Treatment
- Routine Foot Care

Many diabetics develop serious foot problems as a result of poor circulation to the lower extremities (due to hardening of the arteries or atherosclerosis, and neuropathy) resulting in chronic skin ulcers, numbness, and burning of the lower legs and feet. These conditions can be painful and in some cases, particularly when untreated, lead to gangrene, requiring amputation.

Any injury of the feet, in those whose circulation is already compromised, may precipitate infection and delayed healing. The best approach to the problems of the diabetic foot is to prevent the development of foot ulcers with knowledge and prophylactic foot care. It is wise to make sure shoes have adequate toe room to prevent rubbing, which can cause ulcerations or blisters. Soft, well-fitting shoes play an important role in preventing serious foot problems. Diabetics should wear shoes at all times to avoid tiny cuts and splinters that can become infected. Cotton socks are preferable to nylon. Moisturizers may be applied when the feet are dry and talc can be used for excessive perspiration. On the beach, the feet must be covered to avoid sunburn. Swelling and change in color or texture of the foot's skin are significant symptoms and should be followed up promptly by a visit to the family doctor or specialist in diabetes.

Cramps in the leg while walking, particularly of the calf muscle area, may signal the beginning of circulatory problems. The same is true for redness of the feet or darkening of the skin when the legs are in a dependent position. Circulation may deteriorate rapidly causing night pain, which is relieved only by hanging the legs over the side of the bed. "Athlete's foot" must be looked for between the toes and treated with antifungal agents. Poor control of blood sugar interferes with the ability of the white blood cells to fight off infection. Frequent glucose monitoring becomes mandatory in order to ascertain the amounts of insulin required to keep sugar levels near normal.

The foot may become infected, but diabetic neuropathy may mask the pain associated with this serious condition, allowing progression of the process before consultation with a physician is sought. Unless treatment is started promptly, the infection may spread rapidly and gangrenous changes could make amputation a necessity. Charcot's joint, named after a famous French neurologist of the 19th century, results when the neuropathy is severe, causing the ligaments to be damaged and allowing the bones to rub against each other. The bones of the arch of the foot may be unable to maintain their anatomical position and the collapse of the arch results in pressure points and irritation, leading to additional sores and infection. When this ominous chain of events occurs, the patient may require prolonged bed rest for two to four months before healing can take place. In spite of the changes in the feet that prevent ambulation, it is important that the patient continues to use as many muscles as is prudent. This may include arm exercise and upper body movements.

The feet should be inspected before and after any

form of exercise, and instructions from the diabetic educator and permission from your physician must be obtained before embarking on an exercise program. (See Chapter 15, *Benefits of Exercise.*)

When circulation is impaired, it takes longer for sores to heal and makes it easier for infection to develop. The vast majority of the 20,000 foot and leg amputations performed in this country each year can be traced to some degree of neglect. Prevention and attention to minor problems before they become major could help the diabetic population avoid as many as 75% of these devastating procedures.

People who are markedly overweight are more susceptible to foot problems because they cannot reach down to properly inspect their feet for sores, blisters, and infection. Visual problems also may prevent close inspection of the feet in some patients.

Factors That Contribute to the Development
of the Diabetic Foot Ulcer are:

1. Microvascular disease (atherosclerosis) of the small arteries and capillaries supplying oxygen and nutrients to the foot.
2. Damage to nerve tissue (neuropathy), denying the patient awareness of traumatic injuries to the foot from such things as heating pads or carpet tacks.
3. Macrovascular disease (atherosclerosis) of the large vessels causing narrowing and/or blockage of major arteries to the lower legs and feet.
4. Structural deformities, such as hammertoe, cocked toes, bunions, and corns, predispose to the development of ulceration and infection.
5. Poorly fitting shoes can cause undue pressure on the

feet, increasing the risk for calluses or corns. Callus formation is actually a thickening of the outer layers of skin (hyperkeratosis) that causes some loss of cushioning of the bottom of the foot.

Risk factors for peripheral vascular disease include smoking, hypertension, and dyslipidemia. When blood sugar cannot be controlled, elevation of cholesterol and triglycerides occurs, emphasizing the need for strict, proper diabetic management.

PREVENTION OF FOOT ULCERS

The physician must use every means possible to stop any diabetic patient from smoking. Smoking is particularly harmful to the vascular tree. Nicotine constricts the blood vessels, further limiting the circulation. Treating a patient with peripheral vascular disease who smokes is like treating a burn patient while his hand is still in the fire.

Serum lipids must be measured and, if indicated, a rigid low–saturated fat, low-cholesterol diet must be adopted. If lipids still remain elevated, cholesterol-lowering medications can be utilized. (See Chapter 16, *Diabetes, Lipids, and Atherosclerosis.*)

Patients should be taught to examine their feet and toes on a daily basis; checking the spaces between the toes for moisture, and bacterial or fungus infection. Cuts, scratches, blisters, and bruises present potential danger signs. Patients can be taught to examine themselves for decreased feeling, pallor, dryness, or coolness of their lower extremities—signs of impending poor circulation and neuropathy. Molded shoes may prevent formation of bunions, corns, and pressure areas. Infection must be treated promptly.

The feet can be washed gently in lukewarm water, *never hot*. Feet should not be soaked or left in the water, as this softens the skin and makes it more susceptible to maceration and infection. The feet should be dried gently and thoroughly. Moisture-restoring cream should be applied to hold moisture in the skin. Lotions or creams should not be placed between the toes. Talcum powder is used for feet that have a tendency to perspire. (Caution: Do not let the powder cake between the toes.) Toenails should be clipped straight across. Use an emery board to smooth nails. Corns and calluses should never be cut. Ideally, a podiatrist should be consulted for routine foot care, particularly if vision or dexterity are in question. Cotton or wool socks are best for diabetics and should be changed daily. Electric heating pads and hot water bottles have been the culprits in many instances of serious burns to the legs and feet that progressed to gangrene. They must never be used. Debridement of callus formation, trimming, and other forms of foot care should be done by a competent podiatrist, when feasible, rather than by the patient.

When there is evidence of narrowing or blockage of the blood vessels supplying the lower extremities, consultation with a vascular surgeon is in order. Surgical procedures are available to compensate for blockage of involved blood vessels. Vascular bypass operations that shunt blood around the arteriosclerotic vessels are now done routinely. The bypass procedure consists of dissecting out a length of vein from the leg to be used as a shunt around the obstructed artery. An opening is made in the artery below the point of obstruction and the vein is sutured to the artery, end to end. The other end of the vein is reattached to the artery above the point of obstruction, thus serving as a bridge between the unclogged portions of the artery.

Angioplasty is another procedure that is employed to improve the blood flow through blocked arteries. This operation consists of threading a narrow catheter (tube) into the diseased artery until it reaches the point of obstruction. A small balloon at the tip of the catheter is then inflated, exerting pressure against the wall of the vessel and flattening the atheromotous intrusions. The inflation and compression procedure is repeated as required to achieve a sufficiently adequate opening of the vessel to allow a satisfactory blood supply, thus avoiding the more extensive open surgical bypass procedures.

Progression of the ischemia (lack of adequate blood supply), development of infection around the ulcer (cellulitis), and erosion of muscle or bone tissue require immediate hospitalization. To save the extremity may then require the expertise of such specialists as vascular and plastic surgeons and orthopedists.

Treatment of diabetic foot infections can be a therapeutic dilemma due to the difficulties in obtaining accurate bacterial cultures that could serve as a guide for appropriate antibiotic therapy. Infections may spread to bone, causing osteomyelitis, a complication that often proves very difficult to treat.

There are many hospital centers today that specialize in the treatment of diabetic foot ulcers that have achieved marked success in managing infections and saving limbs from amputation. The American Diabetes Association can supply you with the location of nearby centers that can accept referrals from your family doctor or diabetologist. Prompt care can make the difference between saving a limb and disastrous consequences.

It is important to take special care of your feet when you have diabetes. Poor care can lead to serious problems, including foot amputation.

Nerve damage may cause your feet to lose feeling. If this happens, a simple cut or sore can go unnoticed and lead to problems. Nerve damage may change the shape of your feet, causing pressure points. Blisters, sores, and foot ulcers may form in these areas. Poor blood flow to the feet causes injuries to heal more slowly.

One of the most important preventive things you can do is keep your blood sugar as close to normal as is reasonably possible. The Diabetes Control and Complications Trial Study proved that keeping blood sugar as close to normal as possible can reduce the risk of nerve damage by up to 66%.

REVIEW OF FOOT CARE PROCEDURES

Diabetics should be under the care of a podiatrist for routine foot care. If this is not possible, employ the following daily foot care measures.

Daily Foot Care Measures

1. Inspect the feet daily—note the presence of:
    A. Cuts, scratches, bruises, blisters, corns, and calluses
    B. Athlete's foot—especially between the toes
    C. Lack of feeling in the feet
    D. Changes in color of the feet—blue or purple feet may indicate poor circulation
    E. Change in temperature—cold feet may indicate poor circulation
2. Wash feet daily. Bathe, do not soak, feet using warm water and mild soap. Test water temperature with elbow.
3. Dry feet well, especially between toes. You may use a small hand towel for this purpose.
4. For excessively dry feet, apply a good lotion (lanolin, oil, Vaseline) to prevent skin from cracking. Do not apply between toes.

5. When feet sweat, apply a foot powder. If fungus infection develops, use an antifungal powder. Consult with the doctor immediately.

Trimming Toenails

1. Soak feet in basin of warm water for 10–15 minutes. Dry feet well.
2. Use an orange stick to remove debris from under the nail.
3. Trim nails with toenail clipper or special toenail scissors. Cut nails straight across, clipping small sections of the nail at a time.
4. File nails smooth with an emery board or nail file.
5. Do not trim your own nails if your vision or circulation is very poor. Instead, consult with a foot doctor (podiatrist).

Care of Corns and Calluses

1. Keep corns and calluses soft with a lotion.
2. Never use commercial corn removers, razor blades, knives, or household scissors.
3. Consult with a podiatrist if corns and calluses become a major problem.

Treatment of Foot Injuries

1. Wash affected area with soap and warm water.
2. Apply a mild antiseptic—hydrogen peroxide (H_2O_2). Do not use Iodine.
3. If necessary, wrap affected area with sterile gauze or Band-Aid to keep wound clean.
4. Stay off the foot as much as possible to allow it an opportunity to heal. If area becomes red, painful, or

swollen, it is likely to be infected. Consult with your physician *immediately*. Do not wait!

DIABETIC FOOT CARE CHECK LIST

1. Control your diabetes carefully.
2. Keep feet clean and dry.
3. Always protect feet and legs from injury.
   A. Wear clean wool or cotton socks and stockings.
   B. Wear comfortable leather shoes.
   C. Avoid open-toe shoes.
   D. Break new shoes in gradually.
   E. Avoid use of hot water bottles or heating pads, which can burn the skin.
   F. Never walk around barefooted—always wear shoes or slippers.
   G. Never use corn plasters, wart removers, or other over-the-counter foot medications.
4. Promote good circulation.
   A. Avoid smoking. Tobacco in any form produces constriction of the blood vessels.
   B. Do not cross legs at the knees or hook legs around a chair.
   C. Avoid use of restrictive garters, socks, and girdles.
   D. Exercise feet and legs daily. Walking is excellent.

21

Diabetes and Impotence

- Physiologic and Psychologic Causes
- Medical Treatment
- Surgical Treatment

The sexual drive, desire, and performance of diabetic women remains relatively unimpaired even among females with evidence of diabetic neuropathy. The same cannot be said of male diabetic patients, of whom at least 25–35% will develop problems with erection by middle age. The decline in erectile function continues in a steady but often slow fashion and appears *unrelated* to sexual drive or libido. Some studies indicate that up to 50% of diabetic men over the age of fifty will begin to note some difficulty in maintaining an erection and a smaller percentage may experience impotence at an even earlier age. It now appears that adherence to strict diabetic control may lessen the incidence of sexual function difficulties.

Of course, impotence in the Type I or juvenile patient may have a more devastating impact than in the older maturity-onset diabetic, although men of all age groups experience severe psychological stress when this "symbol" of manhood is lost. As in the male population at large, diabetics vary widely in their prediabetic libido, due to the same factors that affect everyone, i.e., emotional stress, depression, marital discord, associated medical problems (cardiac, pulmonary, circulatory, etc.), and as a side effect of medications taken to treat these disorders.

Many people are unaware of the precise definition of impotence. Impotence means the inability to have a firm erection of the penis, sufficient for penetration and the satisfactory achievement of ejaculation. Although erectile dysfunction increases with age, it is not an inevitable consequence of the aging process.

There are many complex physiologic and psychologic functions of the body involved in obtaining and maintaining an erection. One of the most prominent is psychologic. In fact, the mind has been called by some "the most important sexual organ."

Anxiety and depression can occur in the diabetic just as in the non-diabetic and may be confused with organic causes for the failure to achieve a satisfactory sexual relationship.

Endocrine disorders, though rare, can diminish or prevent sexual arousal. For erection to occur, the body's complex hormonal, vascular, neurological, and psychological processes must function in a normal manner. This means that the physician must investigate thyroid, adrenal, and testicular function before attributing the diabetic patient's impotence to neurologic dysfunction.

Erection occurs as a result of the three vascular chambers or cylinders in the penis filling with blood, supplied by the penile artery. This filling produces the enlargement, firmness, and rigidity—the erection—of the male sex organ. Erectile dysfunction occurs when not enough blood is supplied to the penis or when the smooth muscle in the penis fails to relax. If there are pathologic changes in the arteries supplying blood to the penis from arteriosclerosis or other medical or surgical disorders, the blood supply to the penis will be inadequate to cause engorgement and erection cannot be achieved.

Impulses transmitted along nerves to the penis allow the blood to flow into the chambers of the penis, thus the neurologic role becomes highly significant in contributing to the normal formation and maintenance of the erection. Injuries to the pelvic nerve plexus during surgery for prostate cancer can also have a devastating effect on sexual function. Surgical procedures, designed to spare these vital bands of nerve tissue during prostatectomy, can be performed by skilled urologists, lessening the possibility of impotence in this procedure. The pudendal nerve provides sensation from the surface of the penis and may be affected by diabetic neuropathy as well.

In evaluating a diabetic patient, it is important for the doctor to take a complete medical history, including a discussion of sexual function. There are many forms of treatment currently available that can be extremely helpful. The doctor can review the glycohemoglobin level in the blood (discussed in Chapter 8) that serves as a barometer of long-term blood sugar control. As noted, a general medical examination to rule out endocrine or psychologic disorders or neurologic or cardiovascular disease is usually done to be sure there are no other medical conditions that may be contributing to or causing the sexual dysfunction.

Medications such as some used to treat high blood pressure, anxiety or depression, and rheumatic aches and pains are known to sometimes have the side effect of depressing sexual function and the ability to sustain an erection in some patients. Alcohol may also play an important role in diminishing sex drive and contributing to impotence. As Shakespeare noted, "Alcohol doth provoketh the desire but taketh away the performance." Psychedelic and hallucinogenic drugs can have stimulatory as well as depressing effects on sexual function. When all of these factors have been considered and deemed not to be playing a significant role, there are several techniques to determine if the impotence is functional or organic. Some of these techniques rely on the fact that a normal mature man has an average of three to four episodes of erection that take place during dream periods of sleep (nocturnal penile tumescence) of which he is usually unaware.

A gauge can be placed around the penis. If an erection occurs, the gauge will snap, ruling out serious organic pathology.

Observation and monitoring of the penis can also be carried out in a "sleep laboratory," but this is quite costly. Less expensive portable units are available for home use and the results can be interpreted by the patient's diabetic specialist or urologist.

The Doppler Ultrasonographic technique is a very useful diagnostic tool to determine the status of the blood vessels that supply the penis. An ample penile blood supply is a primary prerequisite for an erection to occur. In poorly controlled diabetes, premature atherosclerosis may cause a narrowing and/or blockage of the blood supply to the penis, resulting in an inadequate blood supply to the organ. Evaluation of the vascular status of the penile circulation can make a major contribution to understanding the cause of impotence.

TREATMENT OF IMPOTENCE

Treatment of impotence is recommended only for those individuals who feel that the inability to maintain an erection and participate in sexual activity plays an important role in their life.

About 15% of the adult male population is impotent due to such various causes as vascular disease, prostate cancer, spinal injuries, endocrine problems, neurologic and, of course, psychological inhibitions. Some conditions cause the loss of sex drive to be almost complete—for example, men taking antimale hormone drugs for prostate cancer. Other medical or surgical conditions may only sharply dampen the male's sexual desire.

If the patient has a wife or companion who has retained a normal sexual drive, her mate would take that into consideration before making a decision regarding therapy for impotence. Often, this is a joint determination made by both sex partners before appropriate treatment can begin. Advice and guidance with the diabetologist and urologist should also be sought. At times, psychological counseling can be helpful.

Yohimbine, made from the bark of the Yohimbe tree, is reputed to have aphrodisiac properties. Some patients have reported good results with this medication. Yocon is a medication containing Yohimbine that is available by prescription.

There are several external devices on the market for treatment of impotence that do not involve surgical procedures.

Vacuum constriction is a simple and safe method of treating partial or complete impotence. Vacuum devices actually "pull" blood into the penis. A plastic cylinder is fitted over the penis and air is withdrawn from the cylinder creating a vacuum. A constricting band at the base of the penis keeps the blood from leaving the penis.

There are more than 50,000 of these devices currently in use. An acceptable vacuum system should provide a safety valve to allow rapid release if the patient feels uncomfortable after the constriction is applied.

Injections into the base of the penis with vasodilatory medications have proved to be very effective in achieving erection. Many patients initially find the thought of

.inserting a needle directly into the penis repugnant. But the needle employed is quite small and the injection site at the base of the penis causes no more pain than the discomfort associated with an injection of insulin. However, some lingering pain at the site of the injection is not uncommon. The medication causes the vessels of the penis to dilate, increasing the circulation and reproducing the physiological changes that normally cause erection.

The urologist instructs the patient (and in some cases the partner) in the proper aseptic techniques for these injections. Side effects such as painful persistent erections (priapism), bleeding or bruising, and penile fibrosis (scar tissue) can occur; therefore, frequent consultations with your urologist are necessary.

MUSE URETHRAL SUPPOSITORIES—
A MAJOR THERAPEUTIC BREAKTHROUGH

MUSE (Alprostadil) is a new and unique approach to treating erectile dysfunction. Alprostadil, the active ingredient in MUSE, is identical to a naturally occurring substance found in human semen. Alprostadil has been used for the treatment of erectile dysfunction for many years, and it is well known to physicians for its safety and effectiveness. However, until the development of MUSE, the only way to use Alprostadil was to inject it with a syringe through the skin into the penis. MUSE enables the user to conveniently and quickly administer a therapeutic dose of Alprostadil without the need for injection by inserting a suppository into the urethral opening of the penis. Alprostadil is a vasodilator, meaning it has the pharmacological effect of increasing blood flow to the penis, thereby facilitating erection.

SURGICAL APPROACH

The simplest device for implantation of a penile prosthesis is a semirigid and malleable rod that is permanently implanted in the penis. With this, however, the penis is permanently erect and may require loose-fitting clothing or be bent slightly to avoid embarrassment. These are made of silicone material and the flexibility aids in concealment.

A fully inflatable prosthetic device that more closely simulates erectile function enjoys widespread popularity. This prosthesis consists of expandable penile cylinders that are implanted in the penis, a fluid reservoir implanted in the lower part of the abdomen, and a small pump usually placed within the scrotum. A release valve enables the patient to empty the fluid from the penis after intercourse and the penis returns to its normal flaccid state. The newer designs have solved or greatly improved some of the previous problems with the inflatable penile prosthesis.

Artificial parts for the body considered science fiction a generation ago are now routinely employed. Artificial prostheses of the hip, knee, fingers, and now the male sex organ are routinely employed.

The science of medicine is progressing rapidly. The transplantation of vascular and nerve structures for the benefit of impotence is already being investigated. In the meantime, prosthetic devices are available today for those whose sexual enjoyment and satisfaction contribute greatly to their quality of life.

22

Straight Talk to Teenagers and Young Adults With Diabetes

- What to Tell Friends and Teachers
- How to Live a "Normal" Life
- Answers to Questions Frequently Asked by Young Diabetics

"Oh, you're a diabetic? Don't worry about it. You can live a normal life."

I'll bet you've heard that before. You know better. People mean well when they say, "You can lead a normal life." Maybe they don't realize that you have to take shots of insulin every day. And stick your finger for blood sugar two or three times a day, and say "no thanks" when someone offers you a piece of cake or candy.

The truth is that through no fault of your own, you've got diabetes. The truth also is that you can live a full, productive, and meaningful life.

You're still the same person, with the same personality and the same hopes and ambitions for the future that you have always had. Diabetes can never change that.

Your aim, then, is to manage the diabetes and not let it manage you. There are some questions that will need answers. In this chapter, we answer questions that are frequently asked by friends and family. They mean well, but frankly, most people are misinformed about diabetes and maybe, just maybe, you can enlighten them and make *them* feel more comfortable.

Question 1: What should I tell my friends?
Answer:

Explain that when a person eats, the food is digested and then is broken down and passes into the body's cells to supply energy. This requires a hormone called insulin. Since you don't have enough insulin, you take insulin injections.

It's a good idea to let them know that sometimes your sugar may get too low, causing you to act "shaky and confused." They can help by getting you some sweets or a Coca-Cola, fast.

Question 2: What should I tell my teachers at school?
Answer:

You can tell them the same information you gave your friends. It's a good idea to let them know you may be late on occasions in order to test your blood glucose and to take the proper dose of insulin. It is wise to acquaint the teacher with the symptoms of "low blood sugar" so that she/he can help in an emergency situation. Teachers should be informed about the need for glucose tablets or carbohydrates for treatment of hypoglycemic reactions. Show your teachers and school nurse how to do a blood glucose test and inform them of your target range. There are brochures giving excellent information for teachers that are available through the American Diabetes Association and the Juvenile Diabetes Foundation.

Question 3: Will having diabetes have any effect on my dating?
Answer:

No. Hopefully, you will be with someone who knows your needs and understands the possibility of hypoglycemia or the rare occasion of "running to the bathroom." Your date should be aware of your diabetes and not be surprised by your selection of a proper diabetic diet in a restaurant.

Question 4: Can I participate in sports?
Answer:

As long as you control your blood sugar and monitor it regularly, there are only a very few sports that should be avoided. These would include skydiving, scuba diving, or auto racing. An episode at the wrong time in these sports could cause dangerous problems.

But look what's left: tennis, team sports, biking, swimming, hiking, skiing, and hundreds of other games and activities.

I'm sure you know there have been outstanding stars in major league football, tennis, and baseball, who have had diabetes since childhood. Of course, they are sure to adjust food requirements and insulin dosage before, during, and after strenuous activity. Remember, when you increase physical activity, your insulin and food requirements change. So, plan for this in advance. Contact the International Diabetic Athletes Association for membership and a newsletter.

Question 5: Can I participate at parties?
Answer:

Of course. You can even be the "life of the party."

You are the one who knows what you can eat and how much insulin you must take before going out for the evening. And always have a hard candy or piece of sugar handy, just in case you feel symptoms of low blood sugar. Make sure to check your blood sugar regularly.

Question 6: Will diabetes affect my physical appearance?
Answer:

No. With good diabetic control, your physical development will be right on track. Continue to pay attention to good dental, foot, and skin hygiene, especially around the areas where you give your insulin injections.

Question 7: Will I have difficulty getting a driver's license?
Answer:

No. Usually a doctor's note indicating that your diabetes is under good control is sufficient for the license bureau or state police.

Question 8: Will I be limited in my choice of a career?
Answer:

There are only a few types of work that a person with diabetes would be wise to avoid. This includes jobs that carry a great responsibility for the lives and safety of others, such as a commercial airline pilot, bus driver, or an operator of trains or other public vehicles. I can't think of any other fields that would bar a well-controlled diabetic from participation.

Question 9: What about marriage?
Answer:

There is no reason whatsoever that a diabetic cannot have a long and happy married life. A thorough discussion with your future marital partner should convince you that you have found someone who loves you and can be trusted to be ready to aid you in case some unforeseen diabetic emergency arises. You should be ready to do the same for your future spouse.

Question 10: Will I be able to have children?
Answer:

Modern management has taken away the fear and consternation that existed years ago in regard to pregnancy and fatherhood. With skilled and careful attention to glucose control, there is no contraindication to pregnancy. Remember that it is especially important for the diabetic woman to be well managed *before*, during, and after pregnancy.

Question 11: What about smoking?
Answer:

In this day and age, the general public is now aware of the terrible health consequences of smoking. For the diabetic, it is an absolute no-no. The effect on the lungs, heart, and blood vessels is magnified even more in diabetics. The combination of diabetes and smoking will almost certainly lead to heart and circulatory problems.

Question 12: What about "recreational" drugs?
Answer:

So-called "recreational drugs," such as marijuana, antidepressants, amphetamines, and cocaine, are not only dangerous to your health, but could mask an insulin reaction with all its deleterious consequences. All of these drugs have adverse effects on the diabetic in particular by, in some cases, raising blood sugar, increasing appetite, raising blood pressure, and causing abuse and dependence.

Question 13: What is the effect of alcohol?
Answer:

Alcohol is by far the most addictive drug in general use today in America. While alcohol in small amounts may have a favorable effect on lipids, in larger amounts it can contribute to cardiovascular disease, head and neck cancer, and cirrhosis.

Question 14: What effect does diabetes have on sexual activity?
Answer:

In women, there is little if any effect. In men, good control of blood sugars should allow full sexual activity and enjoyment. Some percentage of men who have had diabetes for many years will develop sexual problems. (This is covered fully in Chapter 21.) Talk to your parents and your doctor or nurse if you have any problems or questions. Sex counts as a physical activity, so you may need an extra snack.

Question 15: What effect do oral contraceptive drugs have on diabetics?
Answer:

It is probably best to avoid "the pill" since it will affect blood sugar, interfere with insulin action, and cause some retention of fluids. Other side effects include high blood pressure and a tendency to form thrombosis (blood clots) in the lower extremities. It is best to seek advice from your physician regarding the best method of birth control for you.

Question 16: Must I continue to test my blood sugar for the rest of my life?
Answer:

The answer to this question is yes. In order to avoid acute and chronic complications of diabetes, blood glucose must be kept within a certain prescribed range. The only way you can do this at the present time is by finger-stick blood sugar determinations. Technical advances are being researched now to obtain blood sugar without the necessity of a finger-stick. We are all hoping this will become available soon.

Question 17: How do I explain to my friends my special needs for injections, glucose monitoring, and meal planning?
Answer:

In a matter-of-fact manner. You will find that people aren't really all that interested and accept you as a person, soon forgetting your special needs. You will still be judged on your merit, conversation, and personality, just as before.

Question 18: Can I look forward to a cure for diabetes?
Answer:

Definitely. Scientists are at work in major medical centers throughout the world attempting to devise new strategies to overcome rejection of islet cell transplants. New medications that one day will "cure" diabetes are the subject of ongoing research. Until then, control your diabetes, retain a bright and cheery outlook, and be optimistic about your future.

Question 19: What can I do to maintain a good management program?
Answer:

Knowledge is power! Learn as much as you can. Put your knowledge about diabetes to use—test your blood glucose regularly, stick to your meal plan, take your medication, and exercise regularly. Enroll in a formal course on diabetes if available. Make sure that you see your doctor for an HbA1c assessment *at least every four months.*

Question 20: Will my insulin requirements change?
Answer:

Probably. Growth, hormone changes with puberty, emotional stress, illness or infection, and changes in exercise may all affect your insulin dose. Write down your blood glucose results so that your doctor can review them and look for patterns. Changes in the patterns of your test results are a signal that adjustments may be needed in your meal plan, insulin dose, or exercise program. (See Chapter 11, *Patterns of Control and Sick Day Care.*)

23

Diabetes in Black Americans

- Epidemiology of Diabetes in African Americans
- Need for Increased Awareness and Treatment
- U.S. Government Conferences

Diabetes mellitus is a major health problem for black Americans. In 1986, the Task Force on Black and Minority Health, appointed by the secretary of the Department of Health and Human Services (DHHS), cited diabetes as one of six health problems responsible for excess mortality among U.S. minority populations.

In 1990, black Americans comprised 12.1% of the U.S. population, according to the U.S. Bureau of the Census. Almost 30 million Americans are black, 13.2% more than in 1980. Census figures document that blacks have higher rates of poverty and unemployment than do whites. They also have a prevalence of non-insulin-dependent diabetes mellitus (NIDDM) that is 60% higher than in whites.

Relatively uncommon among black Americans at the beginning of this century, diabetes is now the fourth leading cause of death by disease among black women and the sixth among black men. A report issued by the National Center for Health Statistics (NCHS) in 1987 noted that the prevalence of diagnosed diabetes in black Americans has increased fourfold in just over two decades, from 228,000 in 1963 to approximately one million in 1985. This is almost double the rate of increase among white, non-Hispanic Americans. Another one million blacks are estimated to have undiagnosed diabetes.

Blacks have higher rates of diabetes at all adult age levels, and among those 65 to 74 years of age, one in four has diabetes. Among black women, diabetes can almost be termed epidemic: One in four black women older than 55 has diabetes—double the rate in white women.

Black Americans also experience higher rates of at least three of the serious complications of diabetes: blindness, amputations, and end-stage renal disease (ESRD). Rates of severe visual impairment are 40% higher in black patients with diabetes than in white patients. Compared to whites, black women are three times more likely to be blind as a result of diabetes and black men have a 30% higher rate of blindness. Black patients undergo twice as many amputations as do whites, and studies in Michigan and Texas found that the rate of ESRD was at least four times higher in blacks with diabetes.

Government surveys indicate that the higher diabetes rate in blacks prevails across all major sociodemographic parameters—age, sex, educational level, marital status, living arrangement, and regional category. The prevalence of diabetes among blacks is highest in women, older people, the less educated, and persons in families with low incomes.

The 1989 National Health Interview Survey (NHIS) queried 600 black Americans and 1,585 white, non-Hispanic Americans with diabetes about various aspects of their diabetes care. Findings reveal that compared to whites, blacks tended to weigh more, were more likely to use insulin and to have received diabetes education, had seen a doctor slightly more often in the past year, and had had their blood pressure and feet checked more often in the past 6 months. In terms of self-monitoring, black patients performed more urine tests each week but fewer blood tests, and they were less likely to have heard of hemoglobin A1c testing.

The NHIS survey also revealed that, compared to whites, a larger percentage of black diabetes patients had seen a dietitian in the past 12 months, and slightly more blacks reported seeing a podiatrist or cardiologist in the past year. Both groups appeared to be comparable in terms of eye care, however. Among both black and white patients, only about 44% had seen an ophthalmologist in the past 12 months, although almost 80% of both black and white patients reported having had an eye examination in the past 3 years. Finally, although black patients were more likely to smoke, they had smoked fewer cigarettes per day than did white patients.

Note: African Americans and Caucasians have the same risk for diabetes at desirable weights. The increased incidence of obesity in the African-American population accounts for the increased incidence of diabetes.

DEFINING THE PROBLEM

The U.S. Government cosponsored two national conferences, one in 1988 and one in 1989, to examine the problem of diabetes in blacks and to define issues and priority areas for activities to reduce the impact of diabetes on black Americans. Both conferences were chaired by Dr. Louis W. Sullivan, secretary of DHHS. The first conference focused on epidemiological and research findings relevant to diabetes and its complications in blacks, and the second on ways to increase diabetes awareness within the professional and black lay communities.

Some major findings noted at the first conference were:

- Black people have a higher prevalence of obesity, a strong risk factor for NIDDM. Among people with diagnosed diabetes, 83% of adult black women are obese compared with 62% of white women, and 45% of black men are obese compared with 39% of white men.
- Black Americans are known to have a high prevalence of hypertension, which is associated with retinopathy and kidney complications, major complications in black patients. Studies are needed to elucidate the disease processes involved in these conditions in black patients and to develop better methods of prevention and treatment.
- Studies of dietary habits of black Americans indicate that they consume less fiber and more cholesterol-rich foods than do whites, although their total intake of calories and fat is lower.
- Black people tend to have less access to financial, social, health, and educational resources that would improve their health status and health awareness.
- Educational resources, including materials and programs oriented to black patients, are needed that take into account black lifestyles, interests, and cultural and economic considerations.

The second conference targeted two critical audiences for diabetes awareness activities: health professionals and the black community itself. Speakers at the conference called for increased physician awareness of diabetes as a serious disease; increased screening activities, especially among high-risk minority patients; and increased education of black patients in modern diabetes management techniques. The need to involve the black community in health promotion activities, especially among black women, was stressed.

The National Diabetes Information Clearinghouse has

compiled a directory of programs and other resources to help health educators, public health officials, community leaders, and others in developing educational programs to foster awareness of diabetes and its management among black Americans. The directory, *Diabetes-Related Programs for Black Americans: A Resource Guide,* includes descriptions of diabetes-related programs that are targeted to black people or that serve communities with substantial black populations. Single copies of the directory are available free from:

National Diabetes Information Clearinghouse
Box NDIC, 9000 Rockville Pike
Bethesda, MD 20892
(301) 468-2162

24

Diabetes in Hispanics

- **High Incidence of Type II Diabetes**
- **Challenge for Hispanics**
- **Spanish Language Publications**

The rate of diabetes among Hispanic Americans, one of the fastest growing minorities in the United States, far exceeds that of white, non-Hispanic Americans. Data from the Hispanic Health and Nutrition Examination Survey (HHANES) of 1982–84 have confirmed what earlier studies have indicated: Diabetes is a major health problem among American Latinos.

Analysis of HHANES data indicates that 1.3 million Hispanics over 21 years of age have diabetes, almost 10% of the adult Hispanic population. Compared with whites, rates of diabetes (diagnosed and undiagnosed) are 50–60% higher in Cubans and 110–120% higher in Mexican Americans and Puerto Ricans.

The most common form of diabetes in Hispanics is non-insulin-dependent (Type II) diabetes, which usually develops in adults over the age of 40. In the 45 to 74 age group, 26.1% of Puerto Ricans, 23.9% of Mexican Americans, and 15.8% of Cubans have diabetes. One-third of Hispanics 65 to 74 years old have diabetes, compared with 17% of non-Hispanic whites in this age group.

Impaired glucose tolerance (IGT), probably the most significant risk factor for diabetes, also is prevalent among older Hispanics. About one-half of Mexican Americans and Puerto Ricans over the age of 55 have either diabetes or IGT, according to HHANES data. Between the ages of 65 and 74, Hispanics are more likely to have abnormal levels of glucose tolerance than normal levels.

Severely overweight Hispanics appear to be at higher risk for diabetes than their non-Hispanic counterparts. Findings from the HHANES study indicate that obese Hispanics, with the exception of Cubans at the highest weight level, are more likely to have diabetes than are obese non-Hispanic whites and blacks. The study also found that among Mexican Americans, 39% of the women and 30% of the men are overweight; among Puerto Ricans, the rates are 37% in women and 25% in men; among Cubans, the rates are 34% in women and 29% in men.

The HHANES is the most comprehensive national survey to date of the health status of Hispanics living on the U.S. mainland. The survey, conducted by the National Center for Health Statistics, included Mexican Americans in five southwestern states, Cubans in the Miami area, and Puerto Ricans in the New York City area.

Other studies in Texas and California indicate that Mexican Americans have higher death rates from diabetes and are more vulnerable to some severe complications of diabetes than are non-Hispanics. In a study conducted in San Antonio, Mexican American diabetes patients had higher rates of severe retinopathy than non-Hispanic patients in that area. These data are confirmed in preliminary findings from a National Health and Nutrition Examination Survey. Other reports suggest that Mexican Americans are six times more likely than non-Hispanics to develop end-stage renal disease, they are more subject to severe hyperglycemia, and Mexican American women have high rates of gestational diabetes and resulting birth complications. Yet, a study of Texas border counties found that 60% of diabetes-caused blindness could have been prevented with proper treatment, as could 51% of kidney failures and 67% of diabetes-related amputations of feet and legs.

The severity of the diabetes problem in Hispanic Americans is compounded by limited access to health care. According to the Current Population Survey of 1989, one-third of Hispanics lack health insurance of any kind, compared with 12% of non-Hispanic whites, about 19% of non-Hispanic blacks, and 18% of other ethnic minorities. Some 37% of Mexican Americans are uninsured, as well as more than 20% of Cubans and 15.5% of Puerto Ricans. Findings from HHANES indicate that uninsured rates among Puerto Ricans and Cubans may be as high as 22 and 28%, respectively. Fewer Puerto Ricans are uninsured because they are more likely to be covered under state Medicaid programs.

The HHANES findings suggest that lack of health insurance may translate into lack of medical care for many Hispanics. The survey shows that uninsured Hispanics were less likely to have seen a physician within the past year and more likely never to have had a physical examination. A study in San Antonio found that uninsured Mexican-American diabetes patients had higher rates of microvascular complications.

These findings pose new problems and considerations for public health programs. Hispanics are currently the second largest minority group in the United States with a population of more than 22 million in 1990. Approximately two-thirds of Hispanics are of Mexican-American origin. Between 1980 and 1990, the Hispanic population grew 40% . By the year 2000, Hispanics may be the largest minority group, with a projected population of 31 million; and by 2080, their numbers may increase an additional 200% (40 million persons).

Hispanics are also a "young" population group, with a median age of about 26 years compared with 34 for the U.S. population as a whole. However, like other population groups, Hispanics are experiencing an increase in life expectancy and their elderly population has increased by 75% since 1980. As the Hispanic elderly population continues to increase, health problems such as non-insulin-dependent diabetes, which is associated with aging, can be expected to have an even greater effect on this community.

Meeting the Challenge: NIDDK Targets Programs for Hispanics

The National Institute of Diabetes and Digestive and Kidney Diseases (NIDDK), the U.S. Government's primary agency for diabetes research, has taken several steps to address the burden of diabetes in Hispanic Americans. In May 1988, Dr. Phillip Gorden, NIDDK director, convened a two-day symposium that brought together leading researchers in the fields of diabetes and Hispanic health care. Speakers discussed characteristics of diabetes and its complications in Hispanics, as well as genetic and non-genetic factors that may account for the higher prevalence of diabetes in this population. Researchers noted that among Mexican Americans in Texas, the risk for diabetes appears to be positively correlated with the degree of Native-American ancestry. Other similarities to diabetes in Native Americans were suggested, including the influence of obesity, particularly upper-body obesity, a westernized lifestyle, and the presence of hyperinsulinism.

The NIDDK supports research projects concerned with diabetes in Hispanics, including projects that address complications of the disorder in this population and projects that focus on primary prevention of diabetes. The

National Eye Institute and the National Heart, Lung, and Blood Institute of the National Institutes of Health have funded research studies in Puerto Rico and Texas on eye and cardiovascular complications of diabetes.

In addition, the NIDDK's National Diabetes Data Group (NDDG) has collaborated with the National Center for Health Statistics in multiple epidemiological surveys that included Hispanic populations. Analysis of data from these surveys is helping NDDG to define more clearly the extent of the diabetes problem in U.S. Hispanics.

The NIDDK has collaborated with the National Coalition of Hispanic Health and Human Service Organizations (COSSMHO) in several projects, including organizing workshops on diabetes for the Sixth Biennial National Hispanic Conference on Health and Human Services and helping to develop an independently funded diabetes research grant program. The Diabetes Research and Training Center at the Albert Einstein School of Medicine in New York City, an NIDDK-funded center, is working with COSSMHO in developing materials for non-Hispanic physicians who care for Hispanic patients.

The National Diabetes Information Clearinghouse (NDIC), a service of NIDDK, distributes a listing of Spanish-language diabetes education materials available from a variety of sources. In addition, the NDIC offers a number of Spanish-language publications, including a dictionary of diabetes-related terms and brochures about periodontal disease and diabetes. These materials are available from:

National Diabetes Information Clearinghouse
Box NDIC, 9000 Rockville Pike
Bethesda, MD 20892
(301) 468-2162

25

The Psychology of Diabetes

- Denial and Rebellion
- Anxiety and Depression
- Effects of Stress
- Family's Role

When one first learns that he has diabetes, he may become confused, depressed, and fearful; and not infrequently, he will enter into a state of denial. Almost everyone has heard the word "diabetes," but like soldiers facing combat who are certain that death or serious injury is something that happens to others, most people feel that they will never have to be concerned with diabetes. The diagnosis often comes as a surprise. Some accept the diagnosis lightly, especially if they feel well and have always considered themselves to be healthy and strong.

These patients prefer to continue life as before, failing to ask questions or to seek guidance in the management of their newly discovered high blood sugar. In their minds, admitting to having diabetes is seen as acquiescing to a threat to their livelihood, a jeopardy to their career, and exposing their vulnerability. It may even arouse sympathy and pity from friends and family. These diabetic patients don't want to learn about "good control" and how to avoid complications. They will often stay on a hypoglycemic pill, usually the first one prescribed, and watch their diet. This is usually interpreted to mean cutting out desserts and not asking for second helpings.

Underneath this facade is a lingering doubt and fear that eventually they will have to follow a stricter diabetic regimen in order to lower the risk of blindness, kidney problems, and a heart attack.

Occasionally, and perhaps for the first time, these patients will hear about a friend or relative with diabetes who has had a heart attack or a stroke at a relatively young age or perhaps early visual changes. This may become the changing point in their lives; they accept the reality of their disease and make the decision to join their doctor in combating their newly detected diabetes.

DENIAL

Others continue in a state of denial and do not seek medical attention until the first sensation of burning and tingling in the toes, a sign of neuropathy, heralds their problem.

Or perhaps they will feel a cramp in the calf muscles while walking. A visit to the doctor elicits a history of frequency of urination and increased thirst and a measurement of the blood sugar above 250 mg/dl. Finally, they will accept the diagnosis and, hopefully, become good patients.

UNDERLYING ANXIETY AND DEPRESSION

Some diabetic patients accept the diagnosis, but maintain an underlying anxiety or depression. They are good patients and accept the advice and guidance of their diabetic educator and physician and attempt to overcome their fears and apprehension. Often, as they realize that they are still the same person, that their life has changed but little, their anxiety and depression is replaced by acceptance of their illness. A desire to adhere to a dietary program emerges; they take their medications or insulin as prescribed and begin a routine of regular exercise with the knowledge that these measures will markedly reduce the risk of future diabetic complications.

WHEN BLOOD SUGAR IS OUT OF CONTROL

Psychological problems arise when glucose levels rise to the point of interfering with concentration, loss of mental alertness, irritability, and depression. These feelings are a direct result of the physiological effect of the elevated blood sugar on the body's metabolism and will subside as the blood sugar is brought under good control.

ROLE OF THE FAMILY

The spouses of diabetics can play an important role once the diagnosis is made. Close family friends will soon know about the patient's diabetes. It is human nature to "spread the news," both good and bad. Members of the family should lend encouragement, join the patient in visits to the diabetic educator, be as familiar with the diabetic diet as the patient, and learn how to handle emergencies should they arise. It is important for the husband, wife, and the children of a diabetic not to become nags—not to constantly remind the diabetic of his condition in regard to monitoring sugar or eating the "right" foods. This type of behavior may only annoy the patient and cause further frustrations contributing to anxiety and depression.

THE PHYSICIAN'S ROLE

The emotional state of the diabetic may depend a great deal on his physician. The doctor should be empathetic, knowledgeable, concerned, and able to motivate the patient in a reassuring manner.

EFFECT OF STRESS

Stress is a part of everyday life. Everyone experiences stress; induced at work, arguments around the house, emotional eruptions with parents or children, or even just watching the television with its constant reminders of crime, corruption, and hate pandering to the very emotions you are trying to keep under control.

The diabetic is more vulnerable to stress because the nervous and endocrine system of everyone, non-diabetic as well as diabetic, reacts to stress by releasing hormones (cortisol, epinephrine, glucagon, and growth hormone) that raise the blood sugar significantly. This can wreak havoc on glucose control. Therefore, avoidance and/or control of stress is very important.

How does one do this? First, if one is a Type A personality—aggressive, "numero uno," the top salesman, or the head of the class—rein in the harness just a little bit and set the sights a little lower. Avoid competing in situations that are not really competitive. You will find you can accomplish the same goals at a slightly slower pace. Don't become a workaholic.

While you should be aware of the lack of integrity and ethics in society today, you should not take the "weight of the world" on your shoulders to correct the world's wrongs. You can join friends and organizations and play a role in helping to improve the relationships between individuals and countries, but keep these endeavors in perspective.

In Chapter 15, *Benefits of Exercise,* the importance of improving all the aspects of metabolism in the diabetic by daily exercise routines was emphasized. Exercise is also an excellent way to relax and relieve stress.

Achieving an occasional break from work and taking vacations when possible will often slow down some of the emotional demons that are contributing to the stressful situations in life. Your doctor may instruct you in the technique of biofeedback, allowing you to control inner tensions and to learn the art of relaxation. For some, yoga, with competent and inspiring instructors, has helped patients to lead a more calm and tranquil life. Frequently, these measures will aid the diabetic to obtain better control of blood sugars in addition to easing the tensions of having to manage a chronic disease.

REBELLION

Rebellion is something that has to be faced, not only in juveniles but also in maturity-onset diabetics. Rebellion can be recognized when the patient refuses to check urine or blood, begins to eat sweets forbidden on the diet program, and refuses to make scheduled visits to the doctor.

Unfortunately, rebellion often ends in the hospital with a severe hypoglycemic attack or ketoacidosis.

When rebellion occurs, the emotional impact on the parents or spouse becomes almost unbearable. If the problem cannot be solved by the cooperation of the physician, the family, and the patient, psychological counseling may be in order.

EFFECT ON PARENTS

When a child is diagnosed as having diabetes, the parents go through a myriad of emotions involving denial, anger, guilt, and despair. Of course, the parents had no control over whether or not their child would develop diabetes. However, when a crisis hits, logic goes out the window. Irrational guilt is common.

After acceptance of the fact that their child has diabetes, parents have to concern themselves with learning about food exchanges, administration of insulin, hygiene, exercise, and all the other components of intelligent diabetic management.

Eventually, the parents learn that with good diabetic control, their diabetic child can live a long and happy life, and with the advances being made every day in the field of diabetic research, a cure may not be too far away. After all, insulin was given to humans for the first time in history only sixty years ago.

WINNING THE BATTLE

The diabetic patient who has overcome the emotional impact of depression and anxiety, who has accepted the fact that he has diabetes and begins intelligent daily management, can take heart in realizing that biomedical research has altered the devastating effects of the acute and chronic complications of diabetes. He should know that diabetics can now live a long, productive, and happy life and that the elimination of this metabolic disease is not too far in the future.

26

Hope for the Future

- Pancreatic and Kidney Transplant
- Islet Cells Transplantation
- Animal Cures
- Newest Drugs
- Genes That Affect Diabetes and Obesity

Researchers continue to search for the cause or causes of diabetes and ways to prevent or cure the disorder. Scientists have found genes that may be involved with NIDDM and IDDM. Some genetic markers for IDDM have been identified, and it is now possible to screen relatives of people with IDDM to see if they are at risk for diabetes.

An ongoing study, The Diabetes Prevention Trial Type I, identifies relatives at risk for developing IDDM and treats them with low doses of insulin in the hope of preventing IDDM. In other words, young people with the potential for the development of IDDM are being treated with low doses of insulin, with the aim of preventing the future development of diabetes. This is a long-term research trial to determine if this therapeutic approach is effective.

There are now signs that while there are many immunologic and technical problems to overcome, these barriers are gradually being surmounted and the promise of a "cure" for diabetes is on the horizon.

One of the major problems confronting successful

transplantation of insulin-producing pancreatic beta cells from donor organs has been the rejection of these "foreign" cells in the diabetic recipient, over a relatively short period of time. The potent immunosuppressive drugs given to avoid rejection are only partially successful and require careful monitoring because of their side effects. It is the rejection process that has frustrated researchers in their search for a permanent cure for Type I diabetes.

Research projects that focus attention on creating tolerance to donor islet cells and reducing or eliminating rejection phenomena are currently underway.

One unique project that has only been carried out in rodents has shown promise in achieving the goal of permanent tolerance to transplanted islets in higher mammals and eventually in human subjects. The thymus is a glandular structure of largely lymphoid tissue, located in the upper anterior chest behind the breastbone. Investigators have shown that by injecting an antigen (a protein or carbohydrate substance that when introduced into the body stimulates the production of an antibody) into the thymus gland, a "tolerance" to the protein develops, and it no longer stimulates antibody production. Organ rejection occurs because no two individuals, with the exception of identical twins, have the same protein components in their cells. When cells from one individual are transplanted to another, the body responds as though a hostile invader has entered its domain. It does not differentiate between an invading bacterium and a transplanted cell. The immune system responds by manufacturing antibodies to seek out and destroy the intruder. Drugs that suppress the immune system—immunosuppresive drugs—are only partially effective in keeping the immunological defense system in check.

Dr. Rodolfo Alejandro of the Diabetes Research Institute of the University of Miami has injected multiple donor islet cells into the thymus gland of rodents and then transplanted them successfully into the kidneys of diabetic rodents. These islet cells functioned normally, manufactured, and released insulin to control the blood sugar of the rodents in response to dietary needs. This transplant procedure induced tolerance that allowed the successful transplantation of insulin-producing islet cells without the inevitability of rejection and without the concomitant use of immunosuppressive drugs. This protocol has not yet been successfully employed in larger animals, and much research remains to be done before rejection problems are overcome.

The concurrent transplantation of bone marrow cells along with islet tissue has produced some interesting results when utilizing the thymus gland as the recipient site. Every time an organ is transplanted, there is a two-way traffic of cells. In this experimental protocol, lymphoid cells go from the recipient into the transplanted islet tissue. From the other direction, transplanted bone marrow cells migrate to other locations in the recipient's body. This phenomenon is called *chimerism*. Much work remains to be done, but further exploration of this phenomenon may turn the key to produce immunological advantage toward tolerance without the use of immunosuppressive drugs.

Many strategies are currently under investigation to render the islet cells nonimmunogenic. The ideal goal is to achieve permanent islet survival by inducing donor tolerance. A novel experimental approach to this problem that shows much promise is the introduction of a semipermeable membrane or microencapsulation coating to isolate the transplanted cells from the immune system of the recipient. This technique has achieved a permanent cure in monkeys. The protective membrane layer or bubble over the transplanted cells permits the free passage of nutrients and wastes, but bars the entrance of antibodies that could destroy the cells. This procedure has resulted in a complete cure of the monkeys so treated, four years after the initial procedure.

Research into the cause, prevention, and cure for diabetes is constantly adding to our knowledge and understanding of the disease. Insulin was first discovered and utilized as a treatment for diabetes at the University of Toronto in 1921 by Banting and Best. In 1996, exciting new pioneering research is being undertaken at Toronto's Hospital for Sick Children. One protocol is based on the fact that Type I diabetes is unknown among the inhabitants of the Samoan Islands, and the only significant difference between their lifestyle and that of their western counterparts is the consumption of animal milk in the diet of western children. It was also noted that in our society, diabetic mothers who breast-fed their offspring reduced the incidence of Type I diabetes in their children by at least two-thirds. The current working hypothesis for this phenomenon is that animal milk contains a peptide—a portion of a protein molecule—that passes into the bloodstream and acts as an antigen to stimulate the production of antibodies against what the body regards as a foreign invader. This milk peptide closely resembles a peptide that occurs naturally in the insulin-producing islet cells of the pancreas. When an allergy to the milk peptide develops, the antibodies produced attack not only the milk peptide but also the individual's own islet cells, which it is unable to distinguish from the offending milk peptide. In this way, the islet cells of the pancreas are gradually destroyed. Type I diabetes is therefore called an autoimmune or self-destructive disease. A large study is currently underway to verify this hypothesis. Three thousand children have been divided into two groups in a double-blind controlled study. One half of them will receive cow's milk and the other half soybean milk or cow's milk that has had the suspected offending peptide altered to render it nonantigenic. This ambitious study will require ten years to give a definitive answer. Although there is much evidence to support this theory, unless a large study is completed, a doubt would always remain as to its validity. Therefore, even though an ethical issue is raised by a study that denies a certain portion of infants of diabetic mothers the theoretical advantage of avoiding cow's milk, the need to know with certainty if the proposed theory for the etiology of Type I diabetes is correct makes the protocol being utilized for this study necessary. The American Academy of Pediatrics has issued an advisory about the possible dangers of cow's milk.

Another approach to prevent or slow down the development of Type I diabetes is being explored in London, Ontario, where investigators are administering Vit. B-3, Nicotinamide, in the belief that this substance will offer protection to the islet cells against autoimmune attack.

We have already discussed the insulin pump that frees patients from rigid eating, sleeping, and exercise schedules and replaces multiple insulin injections with continuous basal and supplemental boluses of short-acting Regular insulin. It is hoped that by skilled use of the pump, one can achieve closer glucose control, prevent or delay or even reverse complications, and permit the diabetic to enjoy a freer lifestyle. The pump has shown beneficial effects on neuropathy, early renal disease, gestational diabetes, and retinopathy. Like the computer and the cardiac pacemaker, we may expect smaller and more easily manageable pumps in the future.

THE "CLOSED LOOP"

The ultimate mechanical device—an "artificial pancreas"—is the "closed loop" system that will incorporate a "glucose sensor" permanently implanted into the patient's vascular system. This conceivably would be able to monitor blood sugar and relay the information to a tiny computerized insulin reservoir that would mete out insulin as required. To be practical, this type of device will require the development of a reliable and fail-safe implantable mechanism. This goal is presently the object of extensive research and development.

TRANSPLANTATION OF THE PANCREAS

In Type I diabetes, the beta cells within the islets of Langerhans are destroyed by repeated autoimmune or viral assaults. While patient self-administration of insulin has altered the prognosis of diabetes to a remarkable degree, in some patients, metabolic control has not been sufficient to prevent the serious by-products of long-standing diabetes, i.e., retinopathy, neuropathy, cardiovascular disease, and nephropathy.

In the past, most recipients of pancreatic transplants would simultaneously undergo kidney transplantation. More recently, with the introduction of more effective immunosuppression drugs, the graft survival rate has improved markedly.

Candidates for simultaneous pancreas and kidney transplant should be between 18 and 55 years of age, free of cardiovascular disease, severe peripheral vascular disease, cancer, or substance-abuse problems.

The indications for pancreas-only transplant have been generally more limited, being restricted to healthier,

younger patients who have unstable (brittle) diabetes without evidence of any severe complications. The surgeon
places the new pancreas in the right side of the patient's
pelvis and attaches it to the corresponding iliac artery and
vein, major vessels that traverse the pelvis. The donor
organ responds like a normal pancreas to the blood sugar
level with appropriate secretion of insulin. A drainage
mechanism is provided by a graft to the bladder for excretion of the digestive enzymes that the transplanted
pancreatic tissue continues to secrete.

Patients must remain on lifelong oral immunosuppressive therapy to prevent rejection of the "new"
pancreas. The failure rate of pancreatic transplants has
been decreasing. The rate of success of combined
pancreas-kidney transplant is about 80% over a five-year
period. The rate for pancreas-only transplants is lower.

Some of the benefits of transplanting the pancreas
are deceleration of diabetic retinopathy, improvement in
cholesterol and triglyceride levels, and improvement of
neuropathy. The patient must remain alert to the side
effects from the immunosuppressive therapy that may
require treatment by his physician.

The transplant of the pancreas or the combined pancreas and kidney is a formidable procedure and performed
only by highly trained, qualified transplant surgeons.

TRANSPLANTATION OF "BETA CELLS" INTO LIVER

Another novel approach, currently the subject of extensive research, involves extracting the tiny "beta cells"
from the pancreas, and after suitable and time-consuming
preparation, injecting them into the portal vein of the diabetic. The hope is that the cells will implant themselves
into the liver and become functional insulin-secreting

tissue. Problems still remain, but the possibility exists that this treatment will become routine in the not too distant future.

NEW DRUGS

Research centers and pharmaceutical companies are continuing their search for newer and better drugs to aid in the control of blood sugar.

Many new medications are in the process of development that will make life easier for the diabetic as we await research to effect a total cure.

In the future, new therapies and drugs to enhance the metabolic actions of insulin, and progress in genetics and gene therapy make the outlook for the diabetic brighter than ever before.

The results of research will one day have a dramatic effect on the lives of millions of diabetics throughout the world. Until then, we must deal with diabetes with our present-day state-of-the art knowledge and discipline.

Glossary

A

ACE Inhibitor A type of drug used to lower blood pressure. Studies indicate that it may also help prevent or slow the progression of kidney disease in people with diabetes.

Acetone A chemical formed in the blood when the body uses fat instead of glucose (sugar) for energy. If acetone forms, it usually means that the cells do not have enough insulin, or cannot use the insulin that is in the blood, to use glucose for energy. Acetone passes through the body into the urine. Acetone is also excreted by the lungs and may cause the breath to smell fruity—"acetone breath." See also: Ketone bodies; ketoacidosis.

Acidosis Too much acid in the body. For a person with diabetes, this can lead to diabetic ketoacidosis. See also: Diabetic ketoacidosis.

Acute Happens for a limited period of time; abrupt onset; sharp, severe.

Adrenal Glands Two organs located on top of the kidneys that make and release hormones such as adrenaline (epinephrine). This and other hormones, including insulin, control the body's use of glucose (sugar).

Adult-Onset Diabetes Former term for non-insulin-dependent or Type II diabetes. See also: Non-insulin-dependent diabetes mellitus.

Adverse Effect A harmful result.

Albuminuria Abnormal amounts of a protein called albumin in the urine. Albuminuria may be a sign of kidney disease, a problem that can occur in people who have had diabetes for a long time.

Alpha Cell A type of cell in the pancreas (in areas called the islets of Langerhans). Alpha cells make and release a hormone called glucagon, which raises the level of glucose (sugar) in the blood.

Amino Acid The building blocks of proteins; the main material of the body's cells. Insulin is made of 51 amino acids joined together.

Amyotrophy A type of diabetic neuropathy that causes muscle weakness and wasting.

Angiopathy Disease of the blood vessels (arteries, veins, and capillaries) that occurs when someone has had diabetes for a long time. There are two types of angiopathy: macroangiopathy, which involves the large blood vessels, and microangiopathy, which involves the small blood vessels.

Antagonist One agent that opposes or fights the action of another. For example, insulin lowers the level of glucose in the blood, whereas glucagon raises it; therefore, insulin and glucagon are antagonists.

Antibodies Proteins that the body makes to protect itself from foreign

253

substances. In diabetes, the body sometimes makes antibodies to work against pork or beef insulins because they are not exactly the same as human insulin or because they have impurities. The antibodies can keep the insulin from working well and may even cause the individual to have an allergic reaction to the beef or pork insulins. See also: Autoimmune disease.

Antigens   Substances that cause an immune response in the body. The body "sees" the antigens as harmful or foreign. To fight them, the body produces antibodies, which attack and try to neutralize the antigens.

Arteriosclerosis   The process by which the walls of the arteries get thick and hard from deposits. In one common type of arteriosclerosis, plaque builds up inside the walls of the vessel. Arteriosclerosis is common in people who have had diabetes for a long time.

Artery   A large blood vessel that carries blood from the heart to other parts of the body. Arteries are thicker and have walls that are stronger and more elastic than the walls of veins.

Aspartame   A man-made sweetener that people use in place of sugar because it has very few calories.

Atherosclerosis   See: Arteriosclerosis.

Autoimmune Disease   Disorder of the body's immune system in which the immune system mistakenly attacks and destroys body tissue that it believes to be foreign. Insulin-dependent diabetes is an autoimmune disease because the immune system attacks and destroys the insulin-producing beta cells.

B

Background Retinopathy   Early stage of diabetic retinopathy; usually does not impair vision. Also called "nonproliferative retinopathy."

Basal Rate   The continuous supply of low levels of insulin, as in insulin pump therapy.

Beta Cell   A type of cell in the pancreas in areas called the islets of Langerhans. Beta cells make and release insulin, a hormone that controls the level of glucose (sugar) in the blood.

Blood Glucose   The main sugar that the body makes from the three elements of food—proteins, fats, and carbohydrates—but mostly from carbohydrates. Glucose is the major source of energy for living cells and is carried to each cell through the bloodstream. However, the cells cannot use glucose without the help of insulin.

Blood Glucose Meter   A machine that tests how much glucose (sugar) is in the blood. A specially coated strip containing a fresh sample of blood is inserted into a machine, which then calculates the correct level of glucose.

Blood Pressure   The lateral force of the blood on the walls of arteries. Two levels of blood pressure are measured—the higher, or systolic, pressure, which occurs each time the heart pushes blood into the vessels, thereby increasing the pressure the blood exerts on the blood vessel wall, and the lower, or diastolic, pressure, which measures the pressure against the wall of the artery when the heart rests between beats. With a blood pressure reading of 120/80, for example, 120 is the systolic pressure and 80 is the diastolic pressure. A reading of 120/80 is said to be the normal range. Blood pressure that is too high is a risk factor for health problems such as heart attacks and strokes.

Bolus An extra boost of insulin given to cover an expected rise in blood glucose such as the rise that occurs after eating.

Borderline Diabetes A term no longer used. See: Impaired glucose tolerance.

Brittle Diabetes A term used when a person's blood glucose (sugar) level often swings quickly from high to low and from low to high. Also called labile or unstable diabetes.

C

C.D.E. (Certified Diabetes Educator) A health care professional who is qualified by the American Association of Diabetes Educators to teach people with diabetes how to manage their condition. The health care team for diabetes should include a diabetes educator, preferably a C.D.E.

C-Peptide A substance that the pancreas releases into the bloodstream in equal amounts to insulin. A test of C-peptide levels shows how much insulin the body is making.

Calcium Channel Blocker A class of drugs used to lower blood pressure.

Carbohydrate One of the three main classes of foods and a source of energy. Carbohydrates are sugars and starches that the body breaks down into glucose (a simple sugar that the body can use to feed its cells). The body also uses carbohydrates to make a substance called glycogen that is stored in the liver and muscles for future use. If the body does not have enough insulin or cannot use the insulin it has, it will be unable to use carbohydrates for energy the way it should. This condition is called diabetes. See also: Fats; protein.

Cataract Clouding of the lens of the eye.

Cerebrovascular Disease Damage to the blood vessels in the brain that may result in a stroke. The blood vessels become blocked because of fat deposits. Sometimes, the blood vessels may burst, resulting in a hemorrhagic stroke. Strokes from a blood clot within the arteriosclerotic vessel are the most common type. People with diabetes are at higher risk for cerebrovascular disease. See also: Macrovascular disease; stroke.

Charcot Foot A foot complication associated with diabetic neuropathy that results in destruction of joints and soft tissue. Also called "Charcot's joint" and "neuropathic arthropathy."

Cholesterol A fatlike substance found in blood, muscle, liver, brain, and other tissues. The body makes and needs some cholesterol. Too much cholesterol, however, may cause a build-up in the artery walls causing arteriosclerosis that slows or stops the flow of blood.

Chronic   Present over a long period of time. Diabetes is an example of a chronic disease.

Circulation   The flow of blood through the heart and blood vessels of the body.

Coma   A sleeplike state; not conscious. May be due to a high or low level of glucose (sugar) in the blood. See also: Diabetic coma.

Complex Carbohydrate   Carbohydrate made up of long chains of sugar, broken down by digestion slowly with less tendency to raise blood sugar than simple carbohydrates.

Complications of Diabetes   Harmful effects that may happen as a consequence of diabetes. Some effects, such as hypoglycemia, can happen any time. Others develop when a person has had diabetes for a long time. These include damage to the retina of the eye (retinopathy), the blood vessels (angiopathy), the nervous system (neuropathy), and the kidneys (nephropathy). Studies show that keeping blood glucose levels as close to the normal, non-diabetic range as possible may help slow, delay, or prevent harmful effects to the eyes, kidneys, and nerves.

Congenital Defects   Problems or conditions that are present at birth.

Congestive Heart Failure   Decreased pumping efficiency and power by the heart, resulting in fluids collecting in the body. Congestive heart failure often develops gradually over several years, although it also can happen suddenly. Generally it can be treated with drugs.

Contraindication   A special condition or circumstance that makes a particular treatment inadvisable.

Controlled Disease   Taking care of oneself so that a disease has less of an effect on the body. People with diabetes can control the disease by staying on their diets, by exercising, by taking medicine if it is needed, and by monitoring their blood glucose. This care will help keep the glucose (sugar) level in the blood from becoming either too high or too low.

Conventional Therapy   A system of diabetes management practiced by most people with diabetes; the system consists of one or two insulin injections each day, daily self-monitoring of blood glucose, and a standard program of nutrition and exercise. The main objective in this form of treatment is to avoid very high and very low blood glucose (sugar). Also called "Standard Therapy."

D

Dawn Phenomenon   A sudden rise in blood glucose levels in the early morning hours. This condition sometimes occurs in people with insulin-dependent diabetes and (rarely) in people with non-insulin-dependent diabetes. Unlike the Somogyi effect, it is not a result of an insulin reaction. People who have high levels of blood glucose in the mornings before eating may need to monitor their blood glucose during the night.

If blood glucose levels are rising, adjustments in evening snacks or insulin dosages may be recommended. See also: Somogyi effect.

Dehydration   Excessive loss of body water. A high level of glucose in the urine causes loss of water by an osmotic excretory effect.

Dextrose   A simple sugar found in the blood. It is the body's main source of energy. Also called glucose. See also: Blood glucose.

Diabetes Control and Complications Trial (DCCT)   A 10-year study (1983–1993) funded by the National Institute of Diabetes and Digestive and Kidney Diseases to assess the effects of intensive therapy on the long-term complications of diabetes. The study proved that intensive management of insulin-dependent diabetes prevents or slows the development of eye, kidney, and nerve damage caused by diabetes.

Diabetic Coma   A major emergency in which a person is not conscious because the blood glucose (sugar) is too low or too high. When the glucose level is too high, the individual has hyperglycemia and may develop ketoacidosis. See also: Hyperglycemia; hypoglycemia; diabetic ketoacidosis.

Diabetic Ketoacidosis (DKA)   Severe, out-of-control diabetes (high blood sugar) with abnormal fat metabolism that needs emergency treatment. DKA occurs when blood sugar levels get too high. This may happen because of illness, taking too little insulin, or getting too little exercise. The body starts using stored fat for energy, and ketone bodies build up in the blood. Ketoacidosis starts slowly and builds up. The signs include nausea and vomiting, which can lead to loss of water from the body, abdominal pain, and deep and rapid breathing. Other signs are a flushed face, dry skin and mouth, a fruity breath odor, a rapid and weak pulse, and low blood pressure. If the person is not given fluids and insulin promptly, ketoacidosis can lead to coma and even death.

Diabetic Retinopathy   A disease of the small blood vessels of the retina of the eye. When retinopathy first starts, the tiny blood vessels in the retina become swollen, and they leak fluid into the center of the retina. The person's vision may then be blurred. This condition is called background retinopathy. If retinopathy progresses, the harm to sight can be more serious. Many new, tiny blood vessels grow out and across the eye. This is called neovascularization. The vessels may break and bleed into the clear gel that fills the center of the eye, blocking vision. Scar tissue may also form near the retina, pulling it away from the back of the eye. This stage is called proliferative retinopathy, and it can lead to impaired vision and even blindness when untreated.

Diabetologist   A doctor who specializes in treating people with diabetes mellitus.

Diagnosis   The term used when a doctor finds that a person has a certain medical problem or disease.

Dialysis   A method for removing waste such as urea from the blood when the kidneys can no longer do the job. The two types of dialysis are: hemodialysis and peritoneal dialysis. In hemodialysis, the patient's blood is passed through a tube into a machine that filters out waste products. The cleansed blood is then returned to the body. In peritoneal dialysis, a special solution is run through a tube into the peritoneal cavity. The peritoneum is a thin tissue that lines the abdominal cavity. The body's waste products are removed through the tube. There are three types of peritoneal dialysis: (CAPD), the most common type, needs no machine and can be done at home. Continuous cyclic peritoneal dialysis (CCPD) uses a machine and is usually performed at night when the person is sleeping. Intermittent peritoneal dialysis (IPD) uses the same type of machine as CCPD, but is usually done in the hospital because treatment takes longer. Hemodialysis and peritoneal dialysis may be used to treat people with diabetes who have kidney failure.

Dietitian An expert in nutrition who helps people with special health needs plan the kinds and amounts of foods to eat. A registered dietitian (RD) has special qualifications. The health care team for diabetes should include a dietitian, preferably an RD.

Dilated Pupil Examination A necessary part of an examination for diabetic eye disease. Special drops are used to enlarge the pupils, enabling the doctor to better visualize the retina for damage.

Diuretic A drug that increases the excretion of fluid from the body. The flow of urine increases as the body rids itself of extra fluid.

DNA (Deoxyribonucleic Acid) A chemical substance in plant and animal cells that contains the genetic formula and tells the cells what to do and when to do it. DNA is the information about what each person inherits from his or her parents. See also: Gene.

Dupuytren's Contracture A condition of the tendons that causes the fingers to curve inward; contraction of the palmar tissue causing permanent flexion of one or more fingers. The condition is more common in people with diabetes and may precede diabetes.

Dyslipidemia Abnormal levels of lipids in the blood.

E

Edema A swelling or puffiness of some part of the body such as the ankles caused by a collection of fluid in the tissues.

Embolus Portion of a blood clot or other substance that becomes detached through the blood until it becomes lodged in a blood vessel, causing obstruction.

Endocrine Glands Glands that produce and release hormones into the bloodstream. They regulate many bodily functions. One endocrine gland is the pancreas. It releases insulin so the body can use sugar for energy. See also: Gland.

Endocrinologist A doctor who specializes in the treatment of problems of endocrine glands. Diabetes is an endocrine disorder. See also: Endocrine glands.

Endogenous Grown or made inside the body. The insulin that is made by a person's own pancreas is endogenous insulin. Insulin that is made from beef or pork pancreas or manufactured is exogenous because it comes from outside the body and must be injected.

End-Stage Renal Disease (ESRD)   The final phase of kidney disease; treated by dialysis or kidney transplantation. See also: Dialysis; nephropathy.

Enzymes   A special type of protein that helps the body's chemistry work better by facilitating chemical reaction.

Etiology   The cause or causes of a certain disease.

Exchange Lists   A grouping of foods by type used with special diets. Each group lists food in serving sizes. A person can exchange, trade, or substitute a food serving in one group for another food serving in the same group. The lists put foods in six groups: (1) starch/bread, (2) meat, (3) vegetables, (4) fruit, (5) milk, and (6) fats. Within a food group, each serving has about the same amount of carbohydrate, protein, fat, and calories. See also: Meal plan.

F

Fasting Blood Glucose Test   A method for determining how much glucose is in the blood when fasting. The test is usually done in the morning after an overnight fast. The normal, non-diabetic range for fasting blood glucose is from 70–110 mg/dl. If the level is over 140 mg/dl (except for newborns and some pregnant women), further evaluation is indicated to make a diagnosis of diabetes.

Fats   One of the three main classes of foods and a source of energy in the body. Fats are the source of vitamins A, D, E, and K. They may also serve as energy stores for the body. In food, there are two types of fats: saturated and unsaturated.

Fatty Acids   A basic unit of fats. When insulin levels are too low or there is not enough glucose to use for energy, the body burns fatty acids for energy. The body then makes ketone bodies, which cause the acid level in the blood to become too high. This in turn may lead to ketoacidosis, a serious problem. See also: Diabetic ketoacidosis.

Fiber   A substance found in foods that comes from plants. Fiber helps intestinal function and is thought to lower cholesterol and help control blood sugar. The two types of fiber in food are soluble and insoluble. Soluble fiber, found in beans, fruits, and oat products, dissolves in water and is thought to help lower blood fats and blood glucose (sugar). Insoluble fiber, found in whole-grain products and vegetables, passes directly through the digestive system, helping to rid the body of waste products.

Foot Care   Taking special steps to avoid foot problems such as sores, cuts, infections, and calluses. Good care includes daily examination of the feet, toes, and toenails, and choosing shoes and socks or stockings that fit well. People with diabetes have to take special care of their feet because nerve damage and reduced blood flow sometimes mean they will have less feeling in their feet than normal and impaired ability to repair tissues. They may not notice cuts and other problems as soon as they should.

Fundus of the Eye   The back or deep part of the eye, including the retina.

Fundoscopy   The visualization of the back area of the eye to see the status of the blood vessels and other conditions that have ocular manifestations. The doctor uses a device called an ophthalmoscope to perform this examination.

G

Gangrene   The death of body tissue. It is most often caused by a loss of blood flow, especially in the legs and feet.

Gene   A basic unit of heredity. Genes are made of DNA, a substance that tells cells what to do and when to do it. The information in the genes is passed from parent to child.

Gestational Diabetes Mellitus   A type of diabetes mellitus that can occur when a woman is pregnant. However, when the pregnancy ends, the blood glucose levels return to normal in about 95% of all cases.

Gingivitis   An inflammation of the gums that, if left untreated, may lead to periodontal disease, a serious gum disease. Signs of gingivitis are inflamed and bleeding gums. See also: Periodontal disease.

Gland   A group of special cells that make substances that help bodily functions. For example, the pancreas is a gland that manufactures insulin, which helps other body cells to use glucose (sugar) for energy.

Glucagon   A hormone that raises the level of glucose in the blood. The alpha cells of the pancreas (in areas called the islets of Langerhans) make glucagon when the body needs to put more sugar into the blood. An injectable form of glucagon, which can be bought in a drug store, is sometimes used to treat hypoglycemia. The glucagon is injected and quickly raises blood glucose levels. See also: Alpha cell.

Glucose   A simple sugar found in the blood. It is the body's main source of energy; also known as dextrose. See also: Blood glucose.

Glucose Tolerance Test   A test to determine if a person has diabetes. The test is given in a lab or doctor's office in the morning before the person has eaten. An initial fasting sample of blood is drawn. The person then drinks a liquid that has a measured amount of glucose (sugar) in it. After one hour, and subsequent intervals, blood samples are taken. The object is to see how well the body deals with a known quantity of glucose in the blood over time.

Gluconeogenesis   The synthesis of glucose from substances that are themselves not carbohydrates, such as protein or fat.

Glycemic Index   Propensity of a food substance to raise the blood sugar. Scientific measurement of blood glucose level response to a food substance.

Glycemic Response   The effect of different foods on blood glucose (sugar) levels over a period of time. Some types of food may raise blood glucose levels more quickly than other foods containing the same amount of carbohydrates.

Glycogen A substance made up of sugars. It is stored in the liver and muscles, and releases glucose into the blood when needed. Glycogen is the chief source of stored fuel in the body.

Glycosuria Having glucose (sugar) in the urine.

Glycosylated Hemoglobin Test A blood test that correlates with a person's average blood glucose (sugar) level for the 2- to 3-month period before the test. See: Hemoglobin A1c.

H

Hemoglobin A1c (HbA1c) The substance formed when glucose becomes attached to hemoglobin molecules. The quantity serves as an indicator of average blood sugar levels for the 8–12 week period prior to the test.

High Density Lipoprotein (HDL) "Good" cholesterol.

HLA Antigens Proteins on the outer part of the cell that help the body fight illness. These proteins vary from person to person. Scientists think that people with certain types of HLA antigens are more likely to develop insulin-dependent diabetes.

Home Blood Glucose Monitoring Testing by the individual at home to determine how much glucose (sugar) is in the blood. Also called self-monitoring of blood glucose. See also: Self-monitoring of blood glucose.

Hormone A chemical produced by special cells and secreted directly into the bloodstream to tell other cells what to do. For example, insulin is a hormone made by the beta cells in the pancreas. When released, insulin enables other cells to use glucose (sugar) for energy.

Humalog Insulin A novel type of insulin with more rapid onset and briefer duration of effect than regular insulin.

Human Insulin Man-made insulins that are similar to insulin produced by the human body. Human insulin has been available since October 1982.

Hyperglycemia Too high a level of sugar in the blood; a sign that diabetes is out of control. Many things can cause hyperglycemia. It occurs when the body does not have enough insulin or cannot use the insulin it does have to turn glucose into energy. Signs of hyperglycemia are thirst, a dry mouth, and a need to urinate often.

Hyperinsulinism Abnormally high levels of insulin in the blood. This term most often refers to a condition in which the body produces too much insulin. This condition is often associated with non-insulin-dependent diabetes.

Hyperlipidemia Abnormally high levels of fats (lipids) in the blood.

Hyperosmolar Coma A coma (loss of consciousness) related to high levels of glucose in the blood and requiring emergency treatment.

A person with this condition is weak from loss of body fluids and electrolytes.

Hypertension   Blood pressure that is above the normal range. See also: Blood pressure.

Hypoglycemia   Too low a level of glucose in the blood. This occurs when a person with diabetes has injected too much insulin, eaten too little food, or has exercised without extra food intake. A person with hypoglycemia may feel nervous, shaky, weak, or sweaty, and have a headache and hunger. Taking small amounts of sugar, sweet juice, or food with sugar will usually help the individual feel better within 10–15 minutes. See also: Insulin shock.

Hypotension   Low blood pressure or a sudden drop in blood pressure. A person rising quickly from a sitting or reclining position may have a sudden fall in blood pressure, causing dizziness or fainting.

I

Immunosuppressive Drugs   Drugs that block the body's ability to fight infection or foreign substances that enter the body. A person receiving a kidney or pancreas transplant is given these drugs to stop the body from rejecting the new organ or tissue. Cyclosporin is a commonly used immunosuppressive drug.

Impaired Glucose Tolerance (IGT)   Blood glucose levels higher than normal, but not high enough to be called diabetes. People with IGT may or may not develop diabetes. Other names (no longer used) for IGT are "borderline," "subclinical," "chemical," or "latent" diabetes.

Implantable Insulin Pump   A small pump placed inside of the body that delivers insulin in response to commands from a hand-held device called a programmer.

Impotence   Loss of ability to function sexually in a male.

Insulin   A hormone that helps the body use glucose (sugar) for energy. The beta cells of the pancreas (in areas called the islets of Langerhans) make the insulin. When the body cannot make enough insulin on its own, a person with diabetes must inject insulin made from other sources, i.e., beef, pork, human insulin (recombinant DNA), or pork-derived, semisynthetic.

Insulin Antagonist   A substance that opposes or fights the action of insulin. Insulin lowers the level of glucose in the blood, whereas glucagon is an antagonist of insulin and raises blood sugar.

Insulin Binding   The process by which insulin attaches itself to something else. This can occur in two ways. First, when a cell needs energy, insulin can bind with the outer part of the cell. The cell then can bring glucose inside and use it for energy. With the help of insulin, the cell can do its work very well and very quickly. Sometimes the body acts against itself. When this happens, the insulin binds with the proteins that are supposed to protect the body from outside substances (antibodies). If the insulin is an injected form of insulin and not made by the body, the body sees the insulin as an outside or foreign substance. When the injected insulin binds with antibodies, it is not available to bind directly to the cell and do its job. See also: Insulin receptors.

Insulin-Dependent Diabetes Mellitus (IDDM) A chronic condition in which the pancreas makes little or no insulin because the beta cells have been destroyed. The body is then not able to use the glucose for energy. IDDM usually comes on abruptly, although the damage to the beta cells may have begun much earlier. The signs of IDDM are a great thirst, hunger, a need to urinate often, and loss of weight. To treat the disease, the person must inject insulin, follow a diet plan, exercise daily, and test blood glucose several times a day. IDDM usually occurs in children and adults who are under age 30. This type of diabetes used to be known as "juvenile diabetes," "juvenile-onset diabetes," and "ketosis-prone diabetes." It is also called Type I diabetes mellitus.

Insulin-Induced Atrophy Small dents that form on the skin when a person keeps injecting a needle in the same spot. They are harmless.

Insulin-Induced Hypertrophy Small lumps that form under the skin produced when a person keeps injecting insulin at the same site.

Insulin Pen An insulin injection device the size of a pen that includes a needle. It can be used instead of syringes for giving insulin injections.

Insulin Reaction Too low a level of glucose (sugar) in the blood; also called hypoglycemia. This occurs when a person with diabetes has injected too much insulin, eaten too little food, or exercised without extra food. Symptoms are hunger, nausea, weakness, nervousness, shakiness, confusion, and sweating. Taking small amounts of sugar, sweet juice, or food with sugar will usually help the person feel better within 10–15 minutes. See also: Hypoglycemia; insulin shock.

Insulin Receptors Areas on the outer part of a cell that allow the cell to join or bind with insulin that is in the blood. When the cell and insulin bind together, the cell can take glucose from the blood and use it for energy.

Insulin Resistance Many people with non-insulin-dependent diabetes produce enough insulin, but their bodies do not respond normally to the action of insulin. This defective response is called insulin resistance; it is one of the major causes of Type II diabetes.

Insulin Shock A severe condition that occurs when the level of blood glucose drops too low. The signs are shaking, sweating, dizziness, double vision, convulsions, and collapse. Insulin shock may occur when an insulin reaction is not treated quickly enough. See also: Hypoglycemia; insulin reaction.

Intensive Management A form of treatment for insulin-dependent diabetes in which the main objective is to keep blood sugar levels as close to the normal range as possible. The treatment consists of three or more insulin injections a day or use of an insulin pump; four or more blood glucose tests a day; adjustment of insulin, food intake, and activity levels based on blood glucose test results; dietary counseling; and management by a diabetes team. See also: Diabetes Control and Complications Trial; team management.

Islets of Langerhans   Special groups of cells in the pancreas. They make and secrete hormones that help the body break down and use food. Named after Paul Langerhans, the German scientist who discovered them in 1869, these cells sit in clusters in the pancreas. There are five types of cells in an islet: beta cells, which make insulin; alpha cells, which make glucagon; delta cells, which make somatostatin; and PP cells and D1 cells, about which little is known.

J

Jet Injector   A device that uses high pressure to propel insulin through the skin and into the body with a needle.

Juvenile-Onset Diabetes   Former term for insulin-dependent or Type I diabetes. See also: Insulin-dependent diabetes mellitus.

K

Ketoacidosis   See: Diabetic ketoacidosis.

Ketone Bodies   Chemicals that the body makes when there is not enough insulin in the blood and fat must be utilized for energy. When the body does not have the help of insulin, the ketones build up in the blood and then "spill" over into the urine as the body attempts to get rid of them. The body can also rid itself of one type of ketone, called acetone, through the lungs. This gives the breath a fruity odor. High ketone levels lead to serious illness and coma. See also: Diabetic ketoacidosis.

Ketonuria   Having ketone bodies in the urine; a warning sign for the development of diabetic ketoacidosis (DKA).

Ketosis   A condition of having ketone bodies build up in body tissues and fluids. The signs of ketosis are nausea, vomiting, and abdominal pain. Ketosis can lead to ketoacidosis.

Kidneys   Two organs in the lower back that clean waste and poisons from the blood. The kidneys are shaped like two large beans, and act as the body's filter. They also control the level of chemicals in the blood such as sodium, potassium, phosphate, chloride, etc.

Kidney Threshold   The blood level above which a substance such as glucose "spills" over into the urine.

L

Labile Diabetes   A term used to indicate that a person's blood glucose level often swings quickly from high to low and from low to high. Also called brittle diabetes.

Lactic Acidosis   The buildup of lactic acid in the body. Body cells make lactic acid when they use glucose (sugar) for energy. The signs of lactic acidosis are deep and rapid breathing, vomiting, and abdominal pain. Lactic acidosis may be caused by diabetic ketoacidosis, or liver or kidney disease. It is also sometimes seen as a side effect from certain medications.

Laser Treatment Using a special strong beam of light of one color (laser) to heal a damaged area. Laser beams are used to heal blood vessels in the eye. See also: Photocoagulation.

Lipid A comprehensive term for fatty acids and cholesterol.

Low Density Lipoprotein (LDL) "Bad" cholesterol.

M

Macrovascular Disease A disease of the large blood vessels that sometimes occurs when a person has had diabetes for a long time. Lipids build up in the walls of the large blood vessels. Three kinds of macrovascular disease are coronary disease, cerebrovascular disease, and peripheral vascular disease.

Markers Genetic signposts on DNA that serve as indicators for the development, or propensity to develop, a condition or disease.

Maturity-Onset Diabetes Former term for non-insulin-dependent or Type II diabetes. See: Non-insulin-dependent diabetes mellitus.

Meal Plan A guide for controlling the amount of calories, carbohydrates, proteins, and fats a person eats. People with diabetes can use such plans as the Exchange Lists to help them plan their meals so that they can keep their diabetes under control. See also: Exchange lists.

Metabolism The term for the way cells chemically change food so that it can be used to keep the body alive. It is a two-part process. One part is called catabolism—when the body uses food for energy. The other is called anabolism—when the body uses food to build or mend cells. Insulin is necessary for the metabolism of food.

Metformin A medication used as a treatment for non-insulin-dependent diabetes; belongs to a class of drugs called biguanides.

Microalbuminuria Small amounts of albumin in the urine affords a measurable method to detect early stages of diabetic nephropathy.

Mg/dl Milligrams per deciliter. Term used to describe how much glucose is in a specific amount of blood. In self-monitoring of blood glucose, test results are given as the amount of glucose in milligrams per deciliter of blood. A fasting reading of 70 to 110 mg/dl is considered in the normal (non-diabetic) range.

Microaneurysm Swelling that forms on the side of tiny blood vessels. These small swellings may break and bleed into nearby tissue. People with diabetes sometimes get microaneurysms in the retina of the eye.

Microvascular Disease Disease of the small blood vessels that sometimes occurs when a person has had diabetes for a long time. The walls of the vessels become abnormally thick, but weak, and therefore they bleed, leak protein, and slow the flow of blood.

Mixed Dose Combining two kinds of insulin in one injection. A mixed dose commonly combines regular insulin, which is fast-acting, with a longer-acting insulin such as NPH. A mixed-dose insulin schedule may be prescribed to provide both short-term and long-term coverage.

Mononeuropathy A form of diabetic neuropathy affecting a single nerve. The eye is a common site for this form of nerve damage. See also: Neuropathy.

Monosaturated Fats Fats that are liquid at room temperature with limited saturation of their chemical chain. They exert beneficial effect on lipid metabolism.

Myocardial Infarction Permanent damage to an area of the heart muscle from a heart attack. This happens when the blood supply to the area of heart muscle is interrupted because of narrowed or blocked blood vessels.

N

Nephrologist A doctor who specializes in the treatment of kidney diseases.

Nephropathy Disease of the kidneys caused by damage to the small blood vessels or to the glomeruli (units in the kidneys that cleanse the blood). People who have had diabetes for a long time may have kidney damage.

Neuropathy Disease of the nervous system. Many people who have had diabetes for a while have nerve damage. The three major forms of nerve damage are: peripheral neuropathy, autonomic neuropathy, and mononeuropathy. The most common form is peripheral neuropathy, which mainly affects the feet and legs. See also: Peripheral neuropathy; mononeuropathy.

NIDDM See: Non-insulin-dependent diabetes mellitus.

Non-Insulin-Dependent Diabetes Mellitus (NIDDM) The most common form of diabetes mellitus; about 90 to 95% of people who have diabetes have NIDDM, also called Type II diabetes mellitus. Unlike the insulin-dependent type of diabetes, in which the pancreas makes no insulin, people with non-insulin-dependent diabetes produce some insulin, sometimes even large amounts. However, either their bodies do not produce enough insulin or their body cells are resistant to the action of insulin (see Insulin Resistance). People with NIDDM can often control their condition by losing weight through diet and exercise. If not, they may need to combine diet with an oral medication and/or insulin and exercise. Generally, NIDDM occurs in people who are over age 40. Most of the people who have this type of diabetes are overweight. Non-insulin-dependent diabetes mellitus formerly was called "adult-onset diabetes," "maturity-onset diabetes," "ketosis-resistant diabetes," and "stable diabetes."

Non-Ketotic Coma See Hyperosmolar Coma.

NPH Insulin Intermediate-acting insulin.

Nutrition   The process by which the body draws nutrients from food and uses them for physiologic activities.

O

Obesity   Excessively corpulent. Extra body fat (20% or more) for their age, height, sex, and bone structure. Extra body fat is thought to be a risk factor for Type II diabetes.

Ophthalmologist   A medical doctor who specializes in the treatment of eye problems or diseases.

Oral Glucose Tolerance Test (OGTT)   A test to determine if a person has diabetes. See: Glucose tolerance test.

Oral Hypoglycemic Agents   Medications taken by mouth that lower the blood glucose level. Sulfonylurea drugs work by causing the pancreas to release more insulin. Amaryl is a third-generation sulfonylurea drug that is insulin sparing—controls blood sugar without any significant increase in insulin. Glucophage and Rezulin also do not cause a rise in insulin levels and therefore when used alone do not cause hypoglycemia. Some of the newer agents decrease insulin resistance.

P

Pancreas   An organ behind the lower part of the stomach that is about the size of a hand. It manufactures insulin. It also makes enzymes that help the body digest food. Scattered throughout the pancreas are specialized areas called the islets of Langerhans.

Peak Action   The time period when the effect of something is at its strongest; such as when injected insulin has the most effect on lowering the glucose (sugar) in the blood.

Periodontal Disease   Gum disease. People who have diabetes are more prone to periodontal disease than people who do not have diabetes.

Peripheral Neuropathy   Nerve damage, usually affecting the feet and legs; causing pain, numbness, or a tingling feeling. Also called "somatic neuropathy" or "distal sensory polyneuropathy."

Peripheral Vascular Disease (PVD)   Disease of the large blood vessels of the extremities (particularly lower extremities). People who have had diabetes for a long time are prone to develop PVD because arteriosclerotic blood vessels in their limbs do not supply adequate blood. The signs of PVD are aching pains in the calf area when walking and relieved by rest, and foot sores that heal slowly.

Photocoagulation   Using a special strong beam of light (laser) to seal off bleeding blood vessels such as in the eye. The laser can also burn away abnormal blood vessels that should not have grown in the eye. The main treatment for diabetic retinopathy.

Plaque   Atherosclerotic deposit of lipids and fibrous tissue in the well of a blood vessel.

Podiatrist   A doctor of podiatry who treats and takes care of feet.

Podiatry The care and treatment of human feet in health and disease.

Polydipsia Excessive thirst that lasts for long periods of time; a symptom of diabetes.

Polyphagia Great hunger; a symptom of diabetes.

Polyunsaturated Fats A type of fat that comes from vegetables. See also: Fats.

Polyuria Having to urinate often; a common symptom of diabetes.

Postprandial Blood Glucose Blood taken 1–2 hours after eating to see the amount of glucose in the blood.

Proinsulin The precursor substance manufactured in the pancreas that is then made into insulin. When insulin is purified from the pork pancreas or beef pancreas, all the proinsulin is not fully removed. When some people use these insulins, the proinsulin can cause the body to react allergically with a rash, to resist the insulin, or even to make dents or lumps in the skin at the site where the insulin is injected.

Prosthesis A man-made substitute for a missing body part such as an arm or a leg; also an implant such as for the hip.

Protein One of the three main classes of food. Proteins are made of amino acids, which are called the building blocks of the cells. The cells need proteins to grow and to mend themselves. Protein is found in many foods such as meat, fish, milk, poultry, and eggs. See also: Carbohydrate; fats.

Proteinuria Protein in the urine. This may be a sign of kidney damage. See also: Microalbuminuria.

Pruritus Itching of the skin; may be a symptom of diabetes.

R

Rebound A swing to a high level of glucose in the blood after having a low level. See also: Somogyi effect.

Receptors Areas on the outer part of a cell that allow the cell to join or bind with insulin that is in the blood. See also: Insulin receptors.

Regular Insulin A type of insulin that is fast acting.

Renal Of or pertaining to the kidneys.

Renal Threshold The blood level above which a substance "spills" over into the urine. This is also called the "kidney threshold," or "spilling point."

Retina The back lining of the eye that senses light. It has many small blood vessels that are sometimes harmed when a person has had diabetes for a long time.

Risk Factor Anything that raises the chance that a person will get a disease. With non-insulin-dependent diabetes, for example, people have a greater risk of getting the disease if they are overweight.

S

Saturated Fat A type of fat that comes primarily from animals and tends to raise cholesterol levels when they are metabolized. See also: Fats.

Secondary Diabetes Conditions (some relatively infrequent) that can produce glycosuria and hyperglycemia. Some examples are pancreatitis, gastrointestinal disorders, renal disease, and certain drugs.

Self-Monitoring of Blood Glucose A method for a person to test how much glucose (sugar) is in the blood. See also: Home blood glucose monitoring.

Somatostatin A hormone made by the delta cells of the pancreas (in areas called the islets of Langerhans). Scientists think it may control how the body secretes two other pancreatic hormones, insulin and glucagon.

Somogyi Effect A swing to a high level of glucose in the blood from an extremely low level, usually occurring after an untreated insulin reaction during the night. The swing is caused by the release of stress hormones to counter low glucose levels. People who experience high levels of blood glucose in the morning may need to test their blood glucose levels in the middle of the night. If blood glucose levels are falling or low, adjustments in evening snacks or insulin doses may be recommended. This condition is named after Dr. Michael Somogyi, who first described this phenomenon. Also called the rebound effect.

Sorbitol A sugar alcohol the body uses slowly. It is used as a sweetener in diet foods. It is called a nutritive sweetener because it has four calories in every gram, just like table sugar and starch. Sorbitol is also produced by the body.

Species Term employed when referring to the source of insulin: whether synthetically manufactured or derived from pork or beef.

Split Dose Division of a prescribed daily dose of insulin into two or more injections given over the course of a day. Also referred to as multiple injections. Many people who use insulin feel that split doses offer more consistent control over blood glucose levels.

Stiff Hand Syndrome Thickening of the skin of the palm that results in loss of ability to hold hand straight. This condition occurs only in people with diabetes.

Stroke Disease caused by damage to blood vessels in the brain. Depending on the part of the brain affected by the loss of blood supply, a stroke can cause a person to lose the ability to speak or move a part of the body such as an arm or a leg. Usually only one side of the body is affected. See also: Cerebrovascular disease.

Subcutaneous Injection Putting a fluid into the tissue under the skin, but above the muscle with a needle and syringe.

Sucrose Table sugar; a form of sugar that the body must break down into a more simple form before the blood can absorb it and take it to the cells.

Sugar A class of carbohydrates that tastes sweet. Sugar is a quick and easy fuel for the body to use. Types of sugar are lactose, glucose, fructose, and sucrose.

Syndrome A set of signs, symptoms, and/or a series of events occurring together that make up a recognized health problem or entity.

Synthetic Insulin   Insulin produced in the laboratory by means of recombinant DNA chemistry.

Systemic   Conditions that affect the entire body. Diabetes is a systemic disease because it involves many parts of the body such as the pancreas, eyes, kidneys, heart, and nerves.

T

Team Management   Diabetes treatment approach in which medical care is provided by a physician, diabetes nurse, educator, dietitian, and behavioral scientist working together with the patient.

Thrombus   A plug that more or less occludes a blood vessel, caused by coagulation of the blood or some of the formed elements of the blood.

Tight Control—a.k.a Intensive Therapy   Type of diabetes control aimed at keeping blood sugars in narrow range close to normal.

Triglycerides   Fat compounds made up of fatty acids and glycerol; the storage form of fat. Transported in blood as very low density lipoproteins (VLDL).

Type I Diabetes Mellitus   See: Insulin-dependent diabetes mellitus.

Type II Diabetes Mellitus   See: Non-insulin-dependent diabetes mellitus.

U

U-100   See: Unit of insulin.

Ulcer   A break in the skin; a deep sore. People with diabetes may get ulcers from minor scrapes on the feet or legs, from cuts that heal slowly, or from the rubbing of shoes that do not fit well. Ulcers are prone to infection.

Ultrasound   A diagnostic test that utilizes sound waves to produce a picture of internal body structures. It is particularly useful for monitoring pregnancy.

Unit of Insulin   The basic measure of insulin, U-100 insulin, means 100 units of insulin per milliliter (ml or cubic centimeter [cc]) of solution. All insulin made today in the United States is U-100.

Unstable Diabetes   A type of diabetes that exhibits wide swings from high to low and from low to high blood sugar. Also called "brittle diabetes" or "labile diabetes."

V

Vaginitis   An infection of the vagina frequently caused by a fungus. This condition may cause itching or burning and may produce a discharge. Women who have diabetes may develop vaginitis more often than women who do not have diabetes.

Index

A

Acarbose, 100–101
Acetohexamide, 96
Ace inhibitor, 158, 191
acromegaly, 15
Adipex P, 136
African Americans, 20, 229–33
alcohol, 24, 95, 169–70
Aldosterone converting enzyme
    inhibitor, 191
Allopurinol (Zyloprim), 95
alprostadil, 219
Amaryl, 97, 267
American Diabetes Association,
    210
American Heart Association, 159
amputations, 205
angioplasty, 157, 209–10
anorectic drugs, 136–39
antibodies, 12
antigen, 246
antioxidants, 149–50, 170
anxiety, 240–41
antabuse effect, 93
atherosclerosis (blood-vessel
    disease), 51, 147–70,
    183–84, 207, 254
Athlete's foot, 206
autoimmune disease, 8
autonomic neuropathy, 175–76

B

"bad" (low-density lipoprotein)
    cholesterol
    see LDL
balloon angiography, 167
Banting, Frederick, 3, 248

Best, Charles, 3, 248
beta-blockers, 95, 158, 192
beta cells, 3, 8, 254
    transplant of, 246–48, 251–52
    with Type I diabetes, 250
bicarbonate, 15
biguanides, 97–99
bilirubin, 23
Black, Samuel, 169–70
blindness, 184–89
blisters, 144–45, 211
blood fats (lipids), 147
blood glucose levels, 86
    impaired tolerance and, 6–7
    and pregnancy, 21
    "spikes" of, 80–81
blood glucose monitoring, 76–83
    diagnosis of diabetes and, 5–7
    frequency of, 113
    glycosylated hemoglobin and,
        78–82
    and infusion pumps, 125–26
    overall benefits of, 76–77
    pregnancy and, 22–23
    procedures for, 77–78
    products used in, 82–83
    recording results, 78, 145
    self-management, 76–83
body weight, 47–48, 54, 119,
    127–28, 162, 192, 207, 267
    and caloric requirements, 130
    overweight persons, 47–48
boluses, 255
Braunwald, Eugene, 168
breathing, difficult, 14
brittle diabetes, 251, 255
bypass surgery, 157, 167, 168, 209

C

Caesarian section, 22
caffeine, 24
calcium channel blocker, 95, 192, 255
calluses, 144–45, 208, 209, 212
calories, and body weight, 130–39
cell receptor, 11–12
carbohydrates, 49, 121, 122–23, 133, 255
  complex, 52–53, 125, 133–34
  label information on, 164
  simple (sugars), 53, 133–34
cardiovascular disease, 46, 166–69, 183–84
carpal tunnel syndrome, 177
cataracts, 187
cellulitis, 210
Charcot foot, 206, 255
chlorpropamide, 93, 96
cholesterol, 48–54, 141, 147–70, 255–56
  HDL (high density lipoprotein), 52, 141, 148, 152–56, 158, 162, 165–66
  LDL (low-density lipoprotein), 148–50, 152–53, 155–59, 162, 165–66, 170
  normal levels, 51
cholestyramine, 100
cigarettes, 147, 150
colestid, 165
coma, 256
  diabetic, 90–91, 257
complex carbohydrates, 1
complications of diabetes, 171–92, 256
confusion, 239
corns, 208
coronary artery disease, 151, 154, 156–59, 169–70
  see also heart disease
corticosteroids, 95
cow's milk, 248–49
Cushings Syndrome, 15
cystitis, 203–204

D

dawn phenomenon, 122
DCCT (Diabetes Control and Complications Trial), 112–16, 120, 121, 188–89, 211, 257
dehydration, 13, 14
denial, 240
dental care, 199–202
depression, 240–41
desfenfluramine, 136
Diabanese, 93, 96
Diabeta, 97
diabetes, 1, 102
  brittle, 251, 255
  causes of, 10
  complications, 9–10, 12–13, 102, 117, 118, 257
  description of, 1–2, 16–18
  diagnosis of, 5–7, 9–11
  early descriptions, 3
  gestational, 19–25
  history of, 2–4
  less common types of, 4
  long-term complications of, 171–92
  number of cases of, 9
  origin of term, 2
  primary, 4
  secondary types of, 4
  symptoms of, 9, 77
  terminology of, 4, 7, 8
  see also Type I diabetes; Type II diabetes
Diabetes Control and Complications Trial
  see DCCT
diabetes pills, 96–101
  see also pills, diabetes
diabetologists, 54, 144, 189, 210, 217, 218, 257
diabetes traveler, 193–97
Diabinese (chlorpropamide), 93, 96
diagnosis of diabetes, 257
  reaction to, 239–44
dialysis, 257–58

Diazoxide (Proglycem), 95
diet, diabetic, 26–30, 118, 127–39,
 158–63, 169–70
 see also food(s); meal planning;
  nutrition
dieting, chronic, 131
Dilantin, 95
diuretics, 130, 158
dizziness, 180
DNA, recombinant, 3, 64, 258
Dobson, Matthew, 2
drugs, 23, 92–101, 110, 111, 130,
 135–38, 149–51, 165–69,
 182, 252
Dymelor, 96
Dyslipidemia, 136, 147, 150,
 156–59, 165, 184, 208, 258

E
eating
 see diet, diabetic; food(s); meal
  planning; nutrition;
  restaurants
Ecotrin, 151
edema, 258
electromyography, 178
emotional response, 214
 to diabetes, 239–44
endocrinologists, 258
endothelium, 149–50
energy, 1, 13
ephedrine, 135
exchange lists, 30–44, 259
exercise, 24, 25, 135, 140–46, 151,
 196–97, 213
 aerobic, 54, 143–44
 benefits of, 140–46, 158
 and blood glucose level, 142–46
 and eating, 129, 144
 and hypoglycemia, 142
 and insulin, 75
 and metabolism, 142
 and the pump, 142
 precautions, 143–44
 recommendations, 54, 135,
  143–44

warning signs, 144, 206–207
eye care, 114
eye problems
 blurred vision, 202
 prevention, 189
 retinopathy, 184–89
 see also vision

F
family, role of, 241
Fastin, 136
fasting plasma glucose, 21
fats, 122, 125–26, 130, 131,
 159–63, 259
 blood (lipids)
  see also cholesterol;
   triglycerides
 cholesterol and, 45–54
 description of, 147–49
 diabetes as affected by, 147
 label information on, 164
 meal planning and, 45–54
 monosaturated, 59
 polyunsaturated, 59, 268
 saturated, 46, 51, 159–64, 268
 tips on reduction of, 59–61
fatty acids, 142, 259
FDA (Food and Drug
 Administration), 135, 136,
 182
feet, 144–45, 181–82
 see also foot care; foot problems
"Fen-Phen," 136
Fenfluramine (Pondamin), 95, 136
fiber, dietary, 49–50, 128–29, 160,
 161, 179, 259
fluvastatin, 166
foam cells, 149
folic acid, 158–59
food(s), 49, 164
 calorie points, 28–29, 40–44
 exchange lists, 28–39, 110–11
 and exercise, 54
 managing diabetes with, 28–29,
  56–61

for preventing hypoglycemia, 144

preparation and selection of, 30

see also meal planning

foot care, 205–13, 259–60

steps in, 211–13

foot doctors (podiatrists), 209

foot problems, 206–11

first-aid treatment of, 212–13

guidelines for management of, 211–13

Framingham study, 147, 154

"French Paradox", 169–70

friends, 227

G

GDM, 20–21, 23–24, 260

gemfibrozil, 166, 169

genetic factors, 12

gestational diabetes, 19–25

gingivitis, 201, 260

glimepiride, 97

glipizide, 96

glossaries of diabetes-related terms, 253–70

glucagon, 85, 119, 197, 260

Glucophage, 97, 267

glucose levels

see blood glucose levels; blood glucose testing

glucose testing strips, 83

glucose tolerance test (GTT), 260

in pregnancy, 21

glucose tolerance, impaired, 23

Glucotrol, 96

Glucotrol XL, 96

glyburide, 97

glycemic index, 53

glycogen, 85, 261

glycosylated hemoglobin test, 78–82, 113, 119, 192, 261

Glynase Press Tabs, 97

"good" (high-density lipoprotein) cholesterol

see HDL

Greeks, ancient, 2

H

HDL, 52, 141, 148, 152–56, 158, 162, 165–66

health-care team

questions for, 222–28

heart, exercise and, 142–43

heart disease, 154–56, 169–70

hemoglobin A, 79

hemoglobin A1c, 78–82, 113, 116, 261

hemoglobin, glycosylated

see glycosylated hemoglobin test

high blood pressure

see hypertension

Hispanics, 234–38

HMG-CoA reductive inhibitors, 166–69

hygiene, 198–204

hypercholeserolemia, 166

hyperglycemia, 95, 144, 261

diabetic ketoacidosis from, 144

drugs and, 95

Hyperosmolar Nonketotic Syndrome, 15–16

hypertension, 190–92, 208, 262

Hypoglycemia, 84–90, 94–95, 105, 116–17, 142, 262

blood glucose levels in, 84

causes of, 87, 88

drugs and, 95

glucagon for, 85

prevention, 88–89

symptoms of, 86–87

I

illness, 104

complications of diabetes due to, 109–11

meal planning during, 102, 109

impaired glucose tolerance, 23

impotence, 214–20

infusion pumps

see insulin infusion pumps

injection, of insulin
   see insulin injection; injection
     devices
insulin(s), 62–75, 117–18, 195–96,
   262
   absorption, 82
   adjustment of, 126
   alcohol and, 70, 72, 73
   animal, 64, 68
   available concentrations, 67
   beef, 64
   basal, 125–26
   biogenetic, 3, 64
   biosynthetic, 3, 64
   brands of, 68–69
   color coding labels, 67, 70
   discovery of, 3
   exercise and, 142
   history of, 2–4
   in foreign countries, 196
   intermediate-acting, 65–66, 88
   long-acting, 72–74, 80, 88
   measurement and injection of,
     70–75
   mixed doses of, 65–74
   mixing in syringe, 72–74
   pork, 64
   preparing and injecting, 70–75
   receptors, 11–12
   resistance to, 11–12, 52
   short-acting, 65, 72–74, 88
   site of injection, 75
   species, 68–69
   see also intensive diabetes
     therapy
insulin-dependent diabetes
   see Type I diabetes
insulin injection, 227, 269
   methods, 72–74
   with mixed insulin, 72–74
insulin pen injectors, 263
insulin pumps, 113, 118, 121–26,
   142, 262
insulin reactions, 90–91, 263
insulin resistance, 263

insulin shock, 263
intensive diabetes therapy, 112–20,
   263–64
   adjusting for low blood sugar in,
     117–18
   children and, 119
   hypoglycemia and, 116–17
   qualifications for, 119
   risks of, 116–17
International Association for
     Assistance to Medical
     Travelers, 194
Ionamin, 136
islets of Langerhans, 3, 264
Isoniazide, 95

J
jaundice, 23
juvenile-onset diabetes, 9, 264
   see Type II diabetes

K
ketoacidosis, diabetic, 10, 13–15,
   21–22, 257
   defined, 13
   from pump failure, 124
   signs and symptoms, 14
   treatment, 14–15
ketones, 13, 21–22, 24, 80, 118,
   264
ketosis, diabetic, 264
kidney problems, 264
   see nephropathy

L
lactic acidosis, 98
Langerhans, Paul, 3
LDL (low-density lipoproteins)
   ("bad") cholesterol, 148–50,
   152–53, 155–59, 162,
   165–66, 170
legal blindness, 185
Lente insulin, 65
Leptin, 132
Lescol, 166
lipase inhibitors, 135

lipids, 147, 149, 154, 156, 169
Liptor, 166
Lopid, 166
lorelco, 165
lovastatin, 166

M

machines for blood glucose testing, 77–78
macrophages, 149
management of diabetes, intensive, 112–20
  home management, 227
  monitoring methods, 76–83
  during pregnancy, 19–25
  during travel, 193–97
meal planning, 26–39, 55–61, 227, 265
  alcohol and, 225–26
  baseline, 26
  goals of, 26
  major approaches to, 26–28
  pregnancy and, 22–23
  travel and, 194–95
  see also food
    weight-loss programs, 127–39
medic-alert medallion, 195
medications, for diabetes, 62–69, 92–101
  see also insulin(s)
menopause, 169
metabolism, 1, 154, 158–59
Metformin, 94, 97–99, 265
Mevacor, 166
microalbuminuria, 191
mciroencapsulation, 247–48
Micronase, 97
microvascular disease, 52
Minkowski, Dr., 2
monitoring of diabetes, 102–11, 118, 226–27, 248–49, 261
  see also blood glucose
    testing; urine testing
monitoring record, 104, 118
  see also record keeping
MUSE, 219

myocardial infarctions (heart attacks), 167, 168, 183–84, 266

N

National Cholesterol Educational Program (NCEP), 153
National Diabetes Data Group (NDDG), 5–7
nephropathy, 113, 114–15, 189–90, 266
neuropathy (nerve disorders), 115
neuropathies, diabetic, 171–83, 206, 266
  types of, 173–77
Nicotinamide, 249
nicotinic acid, 165, 169
non-insulin-dependent diabetes (NIDDM), 4, 8–12, 229, 232, 266
  see Type II diabetes
NPH insulin, 65, 117–18, 266
nutrition, 267
  meal planning, 26–44
  weight-loss programs, 127–39
  see also food

O

obesity, 23, 127–39
ophthalmologists (eye doctors), 188–89, 202, 267
optic nerve, 185
oral contraceptives, 95
oral hypoglycemic agents, 96–101, 267
  alpha-glucosidase inhibitors, 100–101
  appropriate use, 92–93
  biguanides, 97–99
  first generation, 96
  general recommendations, 92–101
  long-acting, 96
  second generation, 96–97
  secondary failure of, 94
  short-acting, 96–97

stress and, 93
sulfonylurea, 92–97
thiazolidinediones, 99–100
third generation, 97
Orinase
    see Tolbutamide
orlistat, 135–36

P
pancreas, 267
    artificial, 250
    islets of Langerhans, 3
    removal of, 2
    transplantation of, 250–51
    see also beta cells
pancreatitis, 4, 15
periodontal disease, 200
patterned glucose rise, method of,
    102–11
penile prostheses, 220
peripheral vascular disease, 208
phenteramine, 136
phenylpropanolimine, 135
pills, diabetes, 96–101
Pima Native Americans, 12
placenta, 21–22
podiatrists, 211, 267
polyunsaturated fats, 268
Pondamin, 136
potassium, 15
Pravachol, 166–68
Pravachol Primary Prevention
    Study, 168
pravastatin, 166, 168
Precose, 100–101
pregnancy, 19–25, 89
    blood sugar testing in, 21
    delivery and, 22
    glycemic drugs and, 23
    monitoring baby's health in,
        22
    monitoring blood glucose in,
        20
    oral agents and, 23
    oral hypoglycemic drugs, 23
    preexisting diabetes and, 19

primary prevention group, 113
Type I diabetes and, 24
weight gain in, 24
    see also gestational diabetes
primary pulmonary hypertension
    (PPH), 137–38
Pritikin, Nathan, 45–46
Probucol, 165
proteins, 268
psychology of diabetes, 239–44
Public Health Service, 194

Q
questions, 222–28
Questran, 165

R
recombinant DNA, 3, 64
Redux, 136
Registered Dietician, 27
regular insulin, 64–65
research in diabetes treatment,
    245–52
retinopathy, 184–89
Rezulin, 99–100, 267

S
salt, 28
saturated fats, 51, 170, 268
Scandinavian Sinvastin Survival
    Study, 167
secondary diabetes, 4
self-monitoring of blood glucose
    (SMBG), 76–83
Semilente insulin, 64–65
serotonin reuptake inhibitors,
    136–38
sexual dysfunction, 180–81,
    214–20
sexual issues, 180–81, 226
    for men, 180–81, 214–20,
        226
    for women, 181, 204, 226
sexual problems, 180–81,
    214–20

male, assistive devices for, 214–20
Shepherd, James, 168
shoes, 205
sick days
  guidelines for, 109–11
  insulin therapy and, 109–10
  meal planning on, 109
simvastatin, 166–67
skin care, 198–99
smoking, 47–48, 147, 150, 151, 192, 202, 208, 213, 225
sodium chloride, 15
Somogyi Effect, 80, 269
Sorbitol, 269
species, 64, 65, 68–69, 269
statins, 166–69
stress, 47, 93, 242–43, 269
Sulfonylureas drugs, 92–97, 267
  1st generation, 96
  2nd generation, 96–97
  3rd generation, 97, 267
syringes, 70, 196

T
teeth, 199–202
  see dental care
thiazolidinediones, 99–100
time zones, 195
toenails
  care of, 212
tolazamide, 96
tolbutamide, 96
Tolinase, 96
travel, 193–97
triglycerides, 46, 154–55
Troglitazone, 99–100
Type I diabetes, 4, 8–11, 16–18, 151, 157, 190, 214, 245, 248–49, 270
  and beta cells, 8
  causes of, 8–9
  development of new treatments for, 245–52

effects of, 8–10
and exercise, 18, 144
and eye examinations, 187
food patterns, 18
insulin patterns, 62
Type II diabetes, 4, 8–18, 98–99, 127, 190, 270
  causes of, 11–12
  development of new treatments for, 245–52
  and exercise, 12, 18, 54
  food management and, 18, 52
  meal plans for, 52
  onset of, 11

U
ulcers, foot, 207–11, 270
Ultralente, 65
urinary tract infections, 202–204
urine
  ketones in, 118
urine testing, 81–82
  for ketones, 144

V
viral infection, 9–10
vision, blurred, 187
vision problems, 184–85, 202
  eye care, 184–89, 202
vitamin C, 150
vitamin E, 149–50
vitreous, 185
von Mering, Dr., 2

W
weight
  see body weight
weight-loss programs, 47–48, 127–39, 141
  exercise in, 54
  healthy food tips and, 55–61
  meal planning and, 54

pills and, 135–39
reasons for, 47–48
women, urinary infections and
    202–204

X
Xenical, 135–36

Y
yohimbine, 218
Yocon, 218

Z
zinc, 3
Zocor, 166

No home should be without . . .

THE COMPLETE GUIDE TO PILLS

Edited and compiled by Brenda Adderly

THE COMPLETE GUIDE TO PILLS
is

• authoritative, easy to use, and totally reliable

• the most up-to-date, comprehensive reference book of its kind, with more than 1,700 of the most commonly prescribed medications listed alphabetically in a unique, consumer-friendly, quick-fact format

• the only mass market guide to prescription medicine created in association with a distinguished panel of physicians from America's top medical schools, including Yale, Harvard, Duke, and Cornell

THE COMPLETE GUIDE TO PILLS
is the reference guide you'll turn to with
complete trust for all your family's
medical needs.

Published by Ballantine Books
Available in your local bookstore.

A nationally recognized asthma specialist offers reassurance and on-the-spot relief . . .

ASTHMA

THE COMPLETE GUIDE TO SELF-MANAGEMENT OF ASTHMA AND ALLERGIES FOR PATIENTS AND THEIR FAMILIES
By Allan M. Weinstein, M.D.

"Essential for every asthma and allergy sufferer's library."
—DR. MICHAEL KALINER
National Institutes of Health

Breathe easier . . .

Look for
ASTHMA